CONCEPTS, COMPOUNDS AND THE ALTERNATIVES OF ANTIBACTERIALS

Edited by **Varaprasad Bobbarala**

Concepts, Compounds and the Alternatives of Antibacterials
http://dx.doi.org/10.5772/59522
Edited by Varaprasad Bobbarala

Contributors

Silvia Ioan, Hassan Ibrahim, Enas El- Zairy, Lucia Pintilie, Biljana Bozin, Neda Gavarić, Nebojša Kladar, Jasna Kovač, Aleksandra Mišan, Sonja Smole Možina, Franz Bucar, Adalberto Pessoa Jr., Angela Faustino Jozala, Letícia Celia De Lencastre Novaes, Joshua Ayoola Obaleye, Varaprasad Bobbarala, Prema Kumari Jonnada, Louis Jesudas

Published by InTech

Janeza Trdine 9, 51000 Rijeka, Croatia

Publishing Process Manager Iva Simcic

Technical Editor InTech DTP team

Cover InTech Design team

First published December, 2015

Printed in Croatia

Additional hard copies can be obtained from orders@intechopen.com

Concepts, Compounds and the Alternatives of Antibacterials, Edited by Varaprasad Bobbarala

p. cm.

ISBN 978-953-51-2232-6

For EU product safety concerns:
IN TECH d.o.o., Prolaz Marije Krucifikse Kozulić 3, 51000 Rijeka, Croatia,
info@intechopen.com or visit our website at intechopen.com.

Meet the editor

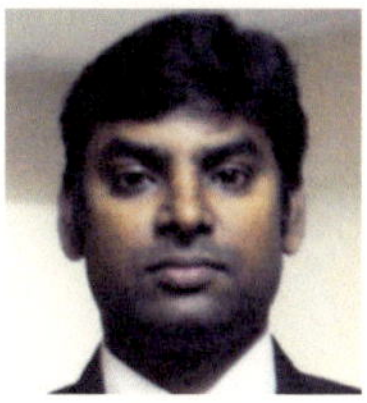

Dr. Varaprasad Bobbarala received his M.Sc. and Ph.D. from Andhra University in 2001 and 2008, respectively. He specialized in Biochemistry, Medicinal Chemistry and Microbiology. He has published over 85 original research articles, reviews and book chapters and edited three books. He is currently the Editor in Chief of the *International Journal of Bioassays* (ISSN: 2278-778X), Associate Editor and member of several editorial boards as well as reviewer of dozens of high-impact international periodicals. Dr. Varaprasad previously served as the Chief Scientist of Research and Development (R&D) at Krisani Innovations Pvt. Ltd., before his current role as the Chief Scientist and Technical Director of Research and Development of Adhya Biosciences Pvt. Ltd., India. He is actively engaged in scientific research in the areas of antimicrobial resistance, isolation of bioactive metabolites and bio-efficacy studies.

Contents

Preface

Antibacterial resistance is spreading globally where bacteria are less- or non-responsive with current antibacterial therapies to prevent bacterial infection, resulting in death and disability of individuals. Infections caused by resistant bacteria often fail to respond to the present-day treatment, resulting in prolonged illness, higher health-care expenditures and a greater risk of death.

According to WHO's 2014 report on global surveillance of antimicrobial resistance, antibiotic resistance is no longer a prediction for the future; it is happening right now, across the world, and is putting at risk the ability to treat common infections in the community and hospitals. Without urging, coordinated action, the world is heading towards a post-antibiotic era, in which common infections and minor injuries, which have been treatable for decades, can once again kill.

In this concern, the present book mainly focuses on the new approaches to better understand antibacterial mechanisms and their mode of action and on searching for environmental alternatives for controlling bacterial pathogens.

Dr. Varaprasad Bobbarala
Chief Scientist
Krisani Innovations Pvt. Ltd.,
Hyderabad, Andhrapradesh,
India

Section 1

The Concepts

Chapter 1

Antibacterial Drugs — From Basic Concepts to Complex Therapeutic Mechanisms of Polymer Systems

Andreea Irina Barzic and Silvia Ioan

Additional information is available at the end of the chapter

http://dx.doi.org/10.5772/60755

Abstract

Infections caused by diverse bacteria represent a major problem that threats the health of humans. This stimulates the scientists to find new solutions for treating these diseases by clarifying the interactions of antibacterial compounds with the biological medium. In this context, the chapter presents some basic concepts regarding the antibacterial drugs. The synthesis routes of novel compounds and specific design techniques with polymer materials are described in correlation with the *in vitro* and *in vivo* activity of antibacterial substances. Essential data about the mechanism of action, selected *in vivo* efficacy and mechanisms of resistance to the most used antibacterial drugs are reviewed.

Keywords: Antibacterial, drugs, classification, synthesis, polymers

1. Introduction

In the past decades, many research findings were directed towards biomedical sciences in an attempt to give a solution to the present health issues caused by microorganism infections. Infectious diseases represent a considerable factor of human morbidity and mortality for most of human existence. The introduction of antimicrobial materials into general clinical use is one of the most successful approaches in chemotherapy, considerably contributing to the control of infections [1]. The existing antimicrobials in the clinical investigations have provided an array of choices when treating many types of infectious diseases. However, treatment options for patients are limited because the bacterial resistance evolved more rapidly than the antibacterial drug development. Clinical results are reporting increasing rates of *in vitro* resistance among previously susceptible organisms and the occurrence of intrinsically resistant microorganisms as pathogens in immunocompromised hosts [2, 3]. To reduce the development and spread of antimicrobial resistance, the preservation of current antimicrobials through their appropriate use becomes mandatory. This motivates scientists to focus on discovery and production of new chemical substances that destroy pathogenic microorganisms with minimal damage to host tissues [4]. Thus, the design of novel classes of antibacterial drugs is redirected on synthesis of compounds with a completely novel mechanism of action [5].

For a deeper understanding of the interactions occurring between the antibacterial drugs and the human beings, in this chapter the basic concepts regarding these bioagents, like definition and classification, are presented. The latter involves the presentation of the main principles, which were taken into consideration to define the effectiveness of an antibiotic. The classical and modern synthesis routes of the main antibacterial drugs are further discussed regarding the main categories of antimicrobial agents. The implications of the preparation methods in designing new therapeutic systems based on polymer materials are analyzed in accordance with the advantages and disadvantages of such delivery devices. A short review on the *in vitro* and *in vivo* activities of antibacterial substances is performed by highlighting the beneficial treatments, and also the secondary effects caused by some delivery systems. Essential data about the mechanism of action, selected *in vivo* efficacy and mechanisms of resistance to the most used antibacterial drugs is presented.

2. Definition and classification of antimicrobial drugs

An antibacterial drug represents a chemical substance derived from a biological source or produced by chemical synthesis that is able to destroy or to inhibit the development/growth of bacteria.

Antibacterial drugs are commonly classified by considering the following criteria:

- **Targeted pathogens:** This category involves antibacterial, antiviral, and antifungal drugs. This grouping may be further subdivided because antibacterial drugs also include urinary antiseptics and anti-mycobacterial drugs. Antimicrobial drugs, especially antibacterial drugs, are strictly classified into chemotherapeutic agents (synthetic chemicals), and antibiotics, produced from living organisms, usually fungi. However, 'antibiotic' is often used loosely to mean all antibacterial drugs;
- **Chemical structure**: Examples are penicillins and cephalosporins;
- **Source**: Natural (mainly fungal sources), semi-synthetic (chemically-altered natural compound), and synthetic (chemically designed in the lab). The "natural" antibiotics arise from fungal sources. Organisms become resistant faster to the natural antimicrobials because they have been pre-exposed to these compounds in nature. Natural antibiotics are often more toxic than synthetic ones. Semi-synthetic drugs appeared as alternative to

http://dx.doi.org/10.5772/60755

decrease toxicity and increase effectiveness of the first category. Synthetic drugs have an advantage that the bacteria are not exposed to the compounds until they are released. They are prepared to exhibit greater effectiveness and less toxicity. There is an inverse relationship between toxicity and effectiveness starting from natural to synthetic antibiotics (Figure 1);

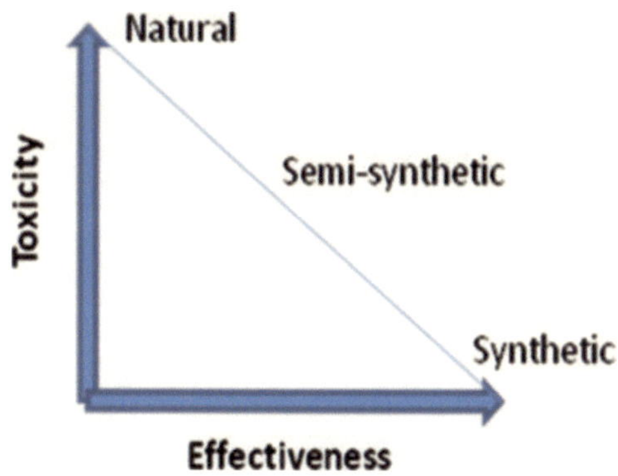

Figure 1. Toxicity *versus* effectiveness for antimicrobial drugs derived from different sources

- Mechanism of action: The antibacterial drugs are designed to have a complex mechanism of action by considering some essential factors which render to the obtained drug-specific features. One can classify antibacterial drugs by taking into account the following:
- *The effect on bacterial growth*
  - bacteriostatic
  - bactericidal drugs
- *The targeted site*
  - drugs that inhibit bacterial wall synthesis or activate enzymes that destroy the cell wall
  - drugs that enhance cell membrane permeability (causing leakage of intracellular material)
  - drugs that determine lethal inhibition of bacterial protein synthesis
  - drugs that generate nonlethal inhibition of protein synthesis
  - drugs that inhibit bacterial synthesis of nucleic acids
  - antimetabolites (disruption of specific biochemical reactions---decrease in the synthesis of essential cell constituents)
  - inhibitors of viral enzymes
- *The target specificity*

- the broad-spectrum drug affects a wide range of disease-causing bacteria, including both Gram-positive and Gram-negative bacteria
- the narrow-spectrum antibacterial drug, which acts against specific families of bacteria. For example, ampicillin is a widely used broad-spectrum antibiotic.

For a better understanding of the different types of antimicrobial drugs, Figure 2 displays the main classes of these substances and their applications.

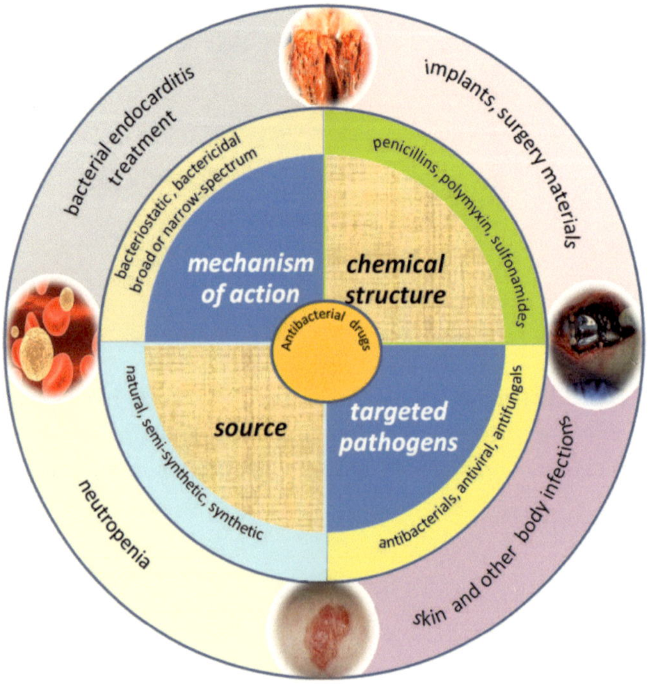

Figure 2. Classification of antimicrobial drugs and their applications

Antibiotics act by inhibiting the basic life-sustaining processes in the microorganism. In order to minimize toxicity, the targets of antibiotics must be selective. However, all antibiotics are toxic to some degree. Selective toxicity should be focused on harming the bacteria, not the host. Selection of the appropriate antibiotic depends on the following parameters:

- Knowledge of organism's natural resistance
- Pharmacological properties of the antibiotic toxicity, binding, distribution, absorption achievable levels in blood, urine
- Previous experience with same species
- Nature of patients underlying pathology
- Patient's immune status

Evaluation of susceptibility focuses mainly on the interaction of antimicrobial agents, the organisms, and their resistance mechanisms. The resistance to antimicrobial drugs is based on several mechanisms, including the following:

- Microbes may generate drug-metabolizing enzymes (such as penicillinase)
- Microbes may cease active uptake of certain drugs
- Microbial drug receptors may suffer change resulting in reduced antibiotic binding and action
- Microbes may produce compounds that antagonize drug actions

Susceptibility tests are essentially artificial measurements that include *in vitro* response, approximate range of effective inhibitory action and reflect possible error equivalent to one tube dilution. The only true measure of bacterial response to an antibiotic drug is the clinical response of the patient (outcome or *in vivo* response).

The bacteria are innately resistant to some antibiotics since they lack a target site or are impermeable to the antibiotic. Resistance spreads between bacteria in three physical ways: conjugation (by direct contact), transduction (by phages), and transformation (uptake of free DNA). The resistance is acquired by spontaneous mutation and conjugation. This could be the results of two aspects as follows:

- Utilization of antibiotics that promote the emergence of drug-resistant microbes
- Suprainfection: A new infection that occurs during the treatment of a primary infection

Delaying the emergence of resistance can be achieved by taking into account the following solutions:

- Use antimicrobial agents only when required
- Utilization of narrow-spectrum antibiotics whenever possible
- Novel antibiotics should be kept for cases in which older drugs are harmful or no longer effective

It is very important that patients should be instructed to strictly follow their prescription particularly during the entire curing treatment period even though symptoms may subside before the full course has been completed. Otherwise, it is possible that interruption of the medication could lead to fail of the treatment and other drugs should be included in the cure. However, there are some disadvantages of antibiotic combinations as follows:

- Enhanced risk of toxic and allergic reactions
- Possible antagonism of antimicrobial effects
- Increased risk of suprainfection
- Selection of drug-resistant bacteria
- High costs

On the other hand, without doctor's advice, the patient might misuse the antibiotics leading to some issues like:

- attempted treatment of untreatable infection (viral infections);
- improper dosage;
- treatment in absence of adequate bacteriologic information
- omission of surgical drainage.

Generally, the prophylactic use of antimicrobial drugs can be divided in three categories: (1) surgery (cardiac, orthopedic, gastrointestinal tract surgery), (2) bacterial endocarditis, and (3) neutropenia. Antimicrobial drugs are also indicated in the treatment of other infections such as young women with recurrent urinary tract infection, prophylaxis against type A influenza with amantadine, lifelong prophylaxis of individuals who have had severe rheumatic carditis. The features of an ideal antibacterial drug are as follows:

- Selective target---target unique
- Bactericidal---kills the bacteria
- Narrow spectrum---does not kill normal flora
- High therapeutic index---ratio of toxic level to therapeutic level
- Few adverse reactions---toxicity, allergy
- Various routes of administration
- Good absorption
- Good distribution to site of infection
- Emergence of resistance is slow

3. Synthesis routes of antimicrobial drugs

The mechanism of action of natural antibacterial agents inspired scientists to prepare more complex structures with improved properties for the cases where the natural products fail due to the resistance occurrence. In this context, the chemical synthesis of new drugs is in continuous evolution. The development of partially or fully synthetic routes to antibacterial compounds is a strategy whose constraints (molecular size and complexity, scalability) must be re-assessed in light of advances in modern chemical synthesis, both strategic and methodological.

Natural products have been a rich source of antibacterial drugs since their discovery, but investments in this domain have been diminished over the past two decades. The main source of natural antibacterial agents is represented by plants, which are able to synthesize aromatic substances, like phenols or their oxygen-substituted derivatives [6]. Most of these substances

http://dx.doi.org/10.5772/60755

are secondary metabolites that serve as plant defense mechanisms against predation by microorganisms, insects, and herbivores. Major classes of antimicrobial compounds obtained from plants are the following:

- Phenolics: simple phenols (catechol, epicatechin), phenolic acids (cinnamic acid), quinines (hypericin), flavonoids, flavones, flavonols, tannins, coumarins
- Terpenoids, essential oils
- Alkaloids
- Lectins and polypeptides
- Polyacetylenes

Catechol is produced industrially by the hydroxylation of phenol using hydrogen peroxide [7]:

$$C_6H_5OH + H_2O_2 \rightarrow C_6H_4(OH)_2 + H_2O$$

This natural antibacterial agent can also be obtained by hydrolysis of 2-substituted phenols, especially 2-chlorophenol, with hot aqueous solutions containing alkali metal hydroxides. Its methyl ether derivative converts to catechol via hydrolysis of the CH_3-O bond as promoted by hydriodic acid.

Terpenoids are prepared by two metabolic pathways:

a. Mevalonic acid pathway

Many organisms manufacture terpenoids through the HMG-CoA reductase pathway, the pathway that also produces cholesterol. The reactions take place in the cytosol.

b. Non-mevalonate pathway

The 2-C-methyl-D-erythritol 4-phosphate/1-deoxy-D-xylulose 5-phosphate pathway (MEP/DOXP pathway), also known as mevalonic acid-independent pathway, occurs in the plastids of plants and apicomplexan protozoa, as well as in many bacteria. Pyruvate and glyceraldehyde 3-phosphate are converted by DOXP synthase to 1-deoxy-D-xylulose 5-phosphate, and by DOXP reductase, (IspC) to 2-C-methyl-D-erythritol 4-phosphate (MEP). The subsequent three-reaction steps catalyzed by 4-diphosphocytidyl-2-C-methyl-D-erythritol synthase (YgbP, IspD), 4-diphosphocytidyl-2-C-methyl-D-erythritol kinase (YchB, IspE), and 2-C-methyl-D-erythritol 2,4-cyclodiphosphate synthase (YgbB, IspF) favor the formation of 2-C-methyl-D-erythritol 2,4-cyclopyrophosphate (MEcPP). Finally, MEcPP is converted to (E)-4-hydroxy-3-methyl-but-2-enyl pyrophosphate (HMB-PP) by HMB-PP synthase (GcpE, IspG), and HMB-PP is converted to isopentenyl pyrophosphate (IPP) and dimethylallyl pyrophosphate (DMAPP) by HMB-PP reductase (LytB, IspH). IPP and DMAPP are the end-products in either pathway, and are the precursors of isoprene, monoterpenoids (10-carbon), diterpenoids (20-carbon), carotenoids (40-carbon), chlorophylls, and plastoquinone-9 (45-carbon). Synthesis of all higher terpenoids proceeds via formation of geranyl pyrophosphate, farnesyl pyrophosphate, and geranylgeranyl pyrophosphate.

Lectins with certain carbohydrate specificity have been purified from various plant tissues and other organisms. On the other hand, these substances can be obtained by recombinant techniques. A sizeable quantity of a lectin (~10g) can result by large-scale fermentation. This procedure is carried out in defined pH value, temperature, optical density at the time of induction, inducer concentration, and time of expression. The most commonly used inducer is isopropyl β-d-thiogalactoside. Subsequently, the cells are harvested by centrifugation. Lectins are released from the cells by resuspension in lysis buffer followed by sonication. Further chromatographic steps are needed for purification of lectins [8]. Isolation of lectins can be accomplished by a combination of several purification techniques. Acids [9], organic solvent, [10] or salt can be used to precipitate lectins. The chromatographic methods, such as affinity chromatography, ionic exchange chromatography, hydrophobic interaction chromatography, and gel filtration are employed. An increase in the number of purification steps usually results in a lesser amount of recovery.

The need for new antibacterial agents remains high, considering the increasing rates of resistance of the drugs available on the market. The results of many of the current therapies with natural products begin to fade, even for common infections.

Semisynthetic antibacterial agents appeared as a result of the researchers efforts to modify the antibacterial substances produced in nature. Thus, semisynthesis came to the forefront of antibacterial discoveries following innovative chemical alterations naturally occurring in some compounds. In the following paragraph, the main chemical insights that helped overcome the numerous limitations of cephalosporin, tetracycline, and macrolide antibacterial drugs, are discussed.

Semisynthesis of β-lactams. It was discovered that cultures of the mold *Cephalosporium acremonium* contained one or more substances that were antagonistic to bacteria. After purification of cephalosporin C from the *Cephalosporium* culture, the 7-aminocephalosporanic acid (7-ACA) is obtained by hydrolysis of cephalosporin C under acidic conditions.

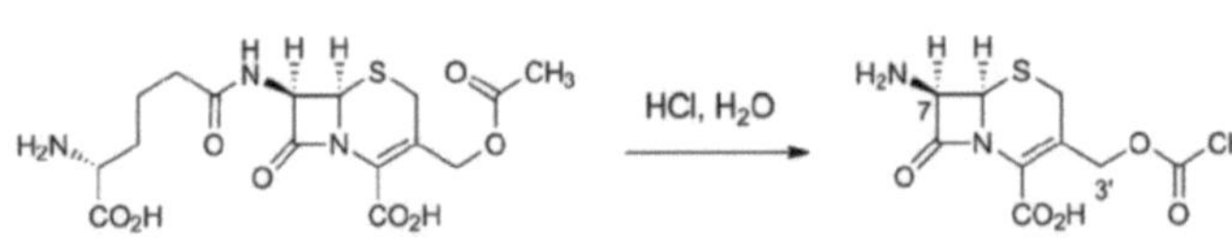

Sheme 1. Hydrolysis of cephalosporin C under acidic conditions

The parenteral cephalosporins (cephalothin) present potent activity against Gram-positive organisms but only moderate activity against Gram-negative bacteria. Improved pharmacological properties, as well as lower susceptibility to resistance mechanisms, are achieved by introducing innovative side chains at just two modifiable sites of 7-ACA---the amine function C7 and C3′.

http://dx.doi.org/10.5772/60755

Semisynthesis of tetracyclines. The development of semisynthetic tetracyclines has been marked by a series of specific, impactful discoveries. The C6-hydroxy group of the natural products oxytetracycline, tetracycline, and 6-demethyltetracycline could be removed reductively. Minocycline was obtained from 6-deoxy-6-demethyltetracycline (sancycline) by an electrophilic aromatic substitution reaction at C7, and it presented a broader spectrum of activity than prior tetracyclines.

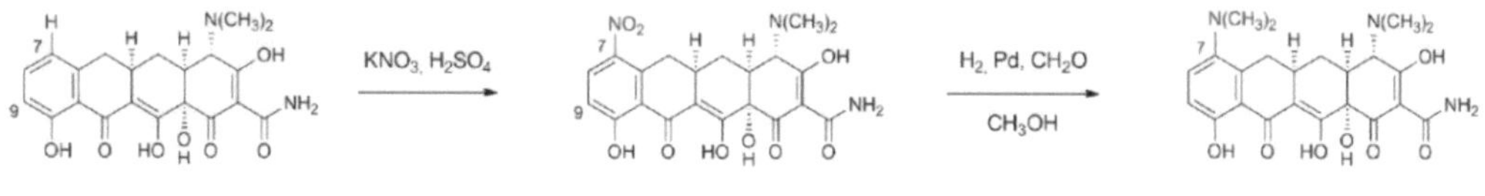

Sheme 2. Preparation steps of minocycline

Semisynthesis of macrolides. Erythromycin, the first macrolide antibiotic (isolated the natural product from the culture broth of the soil-dwelling fungus *Saccharopolyspora erythrea*), is effective against a variety of Gram-positive bacterial infections. However, it possesses poor oral bioavailability and short *in vivo* half-life, and is unstable under acidic conditions, leading to side effects, such as stomach pain. When it is placed in acidic conditions erythromycin decomposes by intramolecular cyclization reactions beginning with addition of the C6 hydroxy group to the C9 ketone, forming anhydrohemiketal and spiroketal derivatives. One solution is to develop a 6-step sequence from erythromycin resulting in selective capping of the C6 hydroxy substituent with a methyl group, affording the antibacterial clarithromycin.

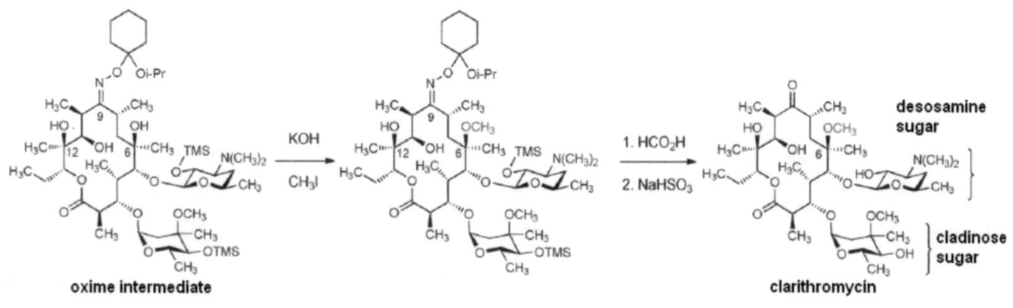

Sheme 3. Preparation stages of clarithromycin

Another innovative semisynthetic solution concerning the chemical instability of erythromycin is focused on removal of the C9 ketone from the erythromycin by a sequence comprising oxime formation, Beckmann rearrangement (ring expansion), and then hydrogenolysis of the iminoether intermediate.

Fully synthetic antibacterial drugs are an alternative solution to the other presented categories. These approaches have also led to important new classes of antibacterial agents and large numbers of approved drugs. The most appreciated examples of synthetic substances used in therapeutics are the chloramphenicol, metronidazole, fosfomycin, quinolones, carbapenems, and oxazolidinones.

Chloramphenicol is a natural compound that is more economical to produce on industrial scale by chemical synthesis rather than fermentation. The substitution of nitro group in chloramphenicol with methanesulfonyl group leads to an increased potency and avoids the fatal aplastic anemia.

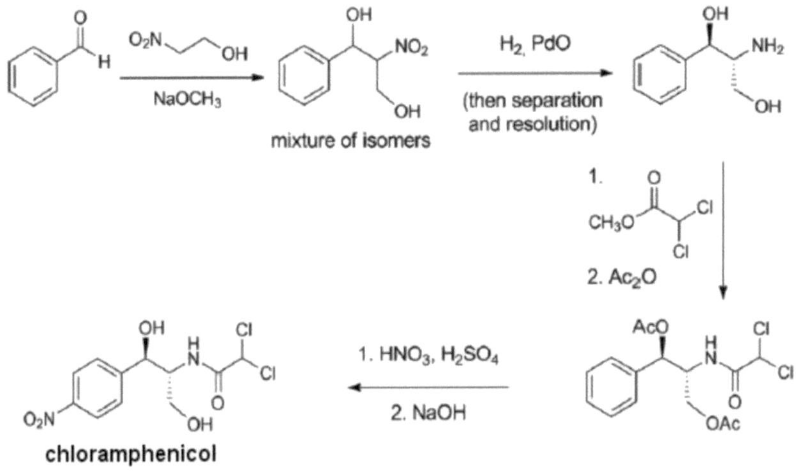

Sheme 4. Synthesis reactions leading to chloramphenicol

Nitroimidazoles (5-nitroimidazole, metronidazole) represent effective drugs for the treatment of trichomoniasis and infections produced by a variety of anaerobic bacteria (including *C. difficile*). 2-Methylimidazole (1) may be prepared via the Debus-Radziszewski imidazole synthesis, or from ethylenediamine and acetic acid, followed by treatment with lime, then Raney nickel. 2-Methylimidazole is nitrated to give 2-methyl-4(5)-nitroimidazole (2), which is in turn alkylated with ethylene oxide or 2-chloroethanol to give metronidazole (3) (http://en.wikipedia.org/wiki/Metronidazole):

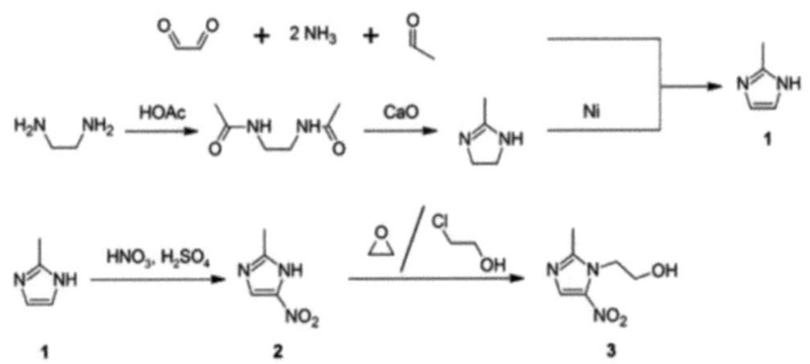

Sheme 5. Preparation steps of metronidazole

http://dx.doi.org/10.5772/60755

Fosfomycin is a polar and small molecule presenting bactericidal activity against both Gram-positive and Gram-negative bacteria due to disruption of cell-wall biosynthesis. This drug prescribed for urinary tract infections is conveniently administered as a single-dose treatment [11]. Fosfomycin was obtained as a secondary metabolite in a glucose-asparagine medium containing citrate for growth and L-methionine combined with L-glutamate for stimulating the production of this compound [12]. More recently, asymmetric synthetic strategy for the synthesis of (-)-fosfomycin was performed using a biocatalytic reduction as the key step [13].

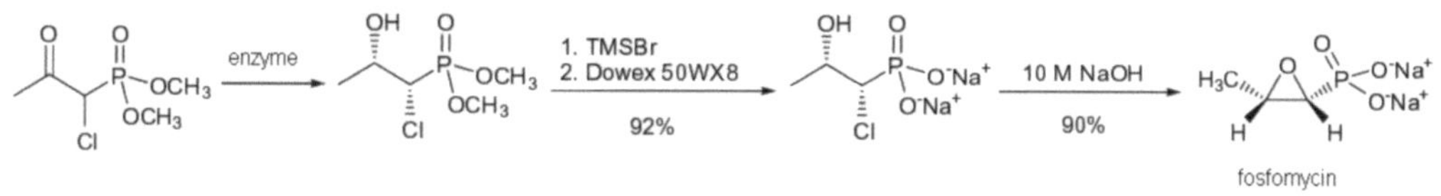

Sheme 6. Synthesis strategy to obtain fosfomycin

Quinolones are more difficult to synthesize in the laboratory than sulfanilamides, but they are obtained by shorter synthetic routes. Norfloxacin is prepared by incorporation of both a fluorine atom at C6 and a piperazine substituent at C7 [8]. The resulted drug presents greatly improved Gram-negative activity and medium activity against Gram-positive bacteria. If the N1 ethyl group of norfloxacin is changed with a cyclopropyl substituent, one obtains ciprofloxacin, which can be used for treatment of respiratory tract, skin, and joint infections, including infections caused by *Pseudomonas aeruginosa.*

Carbapenems arise from the development of fully synthetic β-lactams, leading to a dramatic leap forward in the complexity of antibacterial molecules produced on an industrial scale using fully synthetic approaches. Thienamycin was the first natural "carbapenem" antimicrobial drug. It exhibits exceptional activity against both Gram-positive and Gram-negative organisms, including strains of *Pseudomonas aeruginosa* and organisms with acquired β-lactamase resistance mechanisms. In order to solve the chemical instability problems, it was tried to defer the introduction of the C2-cysteamine side-chain until late in the preparation procedure, enabling a series of analogs with structural variations in the thiol side-chain to be obtained. In the key step of the preparation, the bicyclic carbapenem core is generated in quantitative yield by rhodium-catalyzed cyclization of a diazo-keto ester. This impressive approach led to the discovery of imipenem and other derivatives (obtained by introduction of a C1-β-methyl substituent into the carbapenem core) [14].

Oxazolidinones are active against streptococci and staphylococci. In this class of antibacterial agents, linezolid is the first synthetic compound that helped in curing infections caused by Gram-positive bacteria, like MRSA and vancomycin-resistant enterococci. It is not developed by building upon a naturally occurring skeleton. Several approaches for the synthesis of linezolid have been reported in the chemistry literature [15], but the original preparation procedure developed by Upjohn [15] is lengthy, demands the use of expensive chemicals (palladium on carbon and the highly sensitive reagents methanesulfonyl chloride and n-butyllithium), and needs low-temperature conditions. Later syntheses have included an "atom-economical" method starting from D-mannitol [16] and a route starting from (S)-glyceraldehyde acetonide (prepared from vitamin C) [15]. It was also reported the development of the "second-generation" of linezolid: a convergent, green synthesis starting from (S)-epichlorohydrin, with higher yield and a 56% reduction in total waste [8]. However, long-term use can determine serious adverse effects including bone marrow suppression. Further development of oxazolidinones is based on the x-ray crystal structure of linezolid bound to its target, the large subunit of the bacterial ribosome [17].

A schematic representation of the main synthesis routes of the antibacterial agents is displayed in Figure 3.

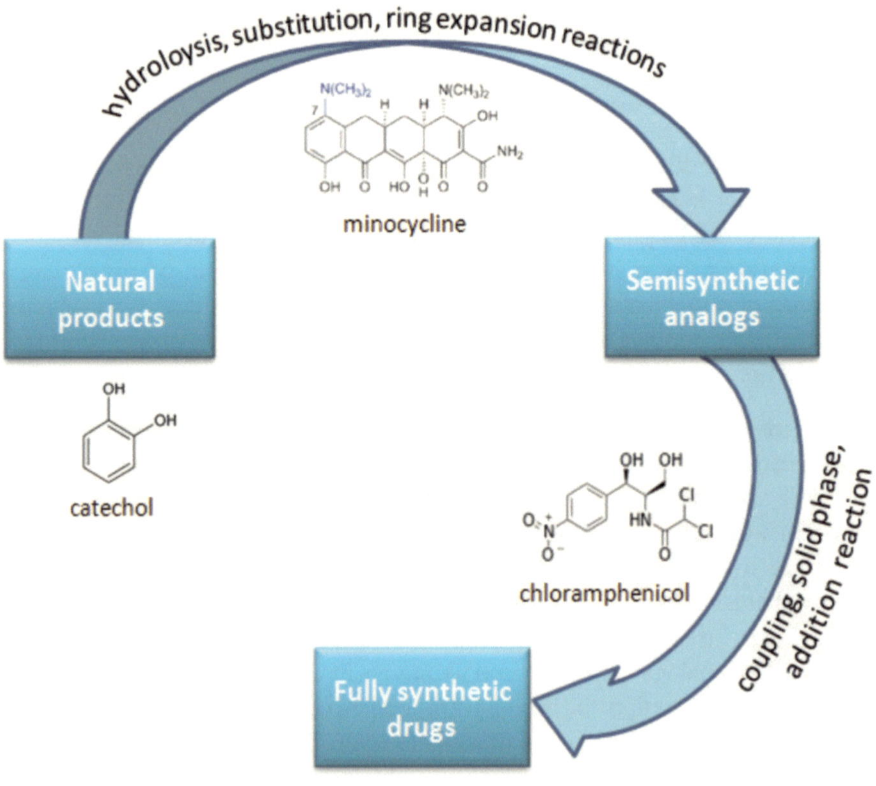

Figure 3. The schematic representation of the main synthesis routes of the antibacterial agents

4. Design of therapeutic systems based on polymers

The design of therapeutic polymer systems with antibacterial action is very complex and it involves special polymerization reactions or chemical functionalization for binding the drugs. Literature reports [18, 19] highlight the influence of some parameters, such as molecular weight, type and degree of alkylation, and distribution of charge on the bactericidal action of antimicrobial polymers. Considering the working principles of antimicrobial macromolecular systems, the design procedures can be divided in three categories (Figure 4), as follows:

- Polymer biocides
- Biocidal polymers
- Biocide-releasing polymers

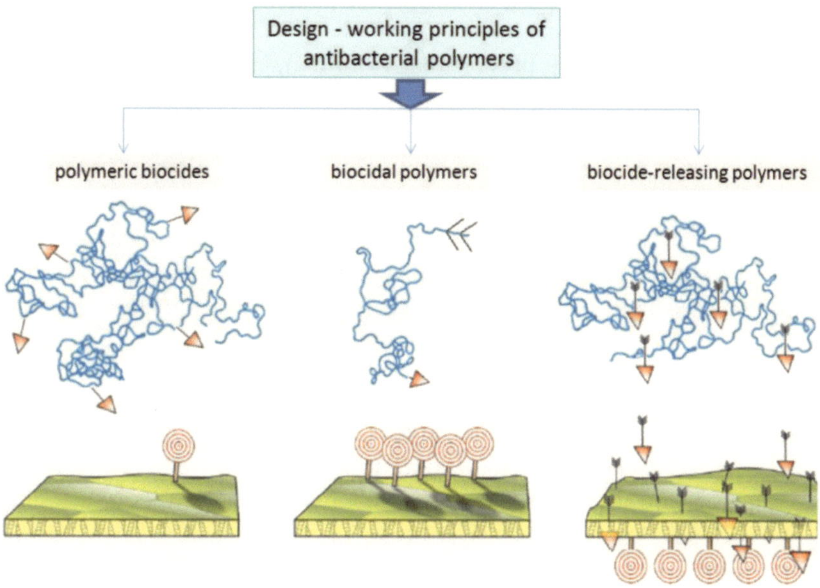

Figure 4. Schematic representation of the design possibilities of antibacterial polymers based on the working principles of macromolecular systems

Polymeric biocides are macromolecules constituted of bioactive repeating units, namely polymers, represent multiple interconnected biocides, which act similarly to the monomers. They can be designed by synthetic routes that yield macromolecules with antimicrobial activity. Their function is not always understood. For instance, polymers and copolymers prepared from 2-methacryloxytroponones are able to kill bacteria. The design of this category of antimicrobial polymers is based on the concept that biocidal groups attached to a polymer act in the same way as analogous low molecular weight compounds, demonstrating that the repeating unit is a biocide. Taking into account the sterical hindrance exerted by the macromolecular backbone, polymeric biocides are expected to be less active than the respective low molecular weight compounds. Literature [20] shows possibility to polymerize antibiotics maintaining their activity at the polymer backbone, e.g., by copolymerization of methacrylate-modified norfloxacin and PEG-methacrylates. Also, polymers with side groups based on hydrophobic quaternary ammonium functions can be considered as polymeric biocides.

The *biocidal polymers* preparation steps require the embodiment of the active principle in the whole macromolecule. It does not necessarily demand the use of antimicrobial repeating units. Microbial cells generally carry a negative net charge at the surface due to their membrane proteins. These charges are prepresented by teichoic acids in case of Gram-positive bacteria, and phospholipids at the outer membrane in case of Gram-negative bacteria. Therefore, polycations are attracted and if they have a proportionate amphiphilic character, they are able to destroy the cytoplasmic membrane, resulting in cell death. The most antimicrobial polycations contain quaternary ammonium [21] and phosphonium [22], tertiary sulfonium [23], and guanidinium functions. Biocidal macromolecules that do not contain biocidal repeating units present antimicrobial activity that originates from the whole molecule. The biocidal repeating units are not required if the polymer backbone exhibits a hydrophobic character. On the other hand, polymers with a hydrophilic polymer backbone demand a hydrophobic region parallel to the backbone, which is provided by the hydrophobic side groups. Polymeric biocides are efficient when cationic groups are placed along the polymer backbone, but the good results are obtained also for polymers having only one biocidal end group. These polymers are obtained by cationic ring-opening polymerization of 2-alkyl-1,3-oxazolines and terminating the macromolecule with a cationic surfactant. The advantage of this preparation technique is the controlled introduction of a specific group at one end and another group at the opposite end of the macromolecules by selecting a suitable initiator and termination agent.

Biocide-releasing polymers do not act through the actual polymeric part, but the latter represents a carrier for biocides that are transferred through different mechanisms (like diffusion) to the infected area. Such polymers are usually the most active systems, because they can release their biocides close to the cell in high local concentrations. The biocide-releasing macromolecules were prepared for the first time through polymerization of salicylic acid subjected to degradation, which enables the controlled releasing of salicylic acid. Several types of biocidal polymers have been designed to release chlorine, nitric oxide, phenols, or singlet oxygen. Another class of biocide-releasing polymers is the contact-active ones, like tributyltin esters of polyacrylates.

Natural polymers, such as collagen, can serve as antibacterial drug carrier. The latter can be complexed to the polymer through direct binding of the biocide to free amino or carboxylic groups of the collagen molecule [24]. The diffusion is the main process that assures the release of the drug after implantation or injection. The design of the sponge and the drug incorporation by colyophilization allow the uniform distribution of the drug within the spongy matrix. This also ensures an equal drug dose applied per square centimeter of the treated surface. Pore size of natural polymer sponges can be controlled by the lyophilization process [24].

On the other hand, synthetic copolymers, like epoxy-functional poly(dimethylsiloxane) can be processed to favor the attachment (i.e., tethering) of levofloxacin [25]. The reaction occurred via ring-opening of epoxy groups by the carboxylic acid group of levofloxacin, the tether produced was an ester-functional tether. Compared to a control coating generated by simply blending levofloxacin into a polysiloxane, the samples with tethered levofloxacin moieties presented uniform distribution of levofloxacin, higher initial kill, and sustained antimicrobial surface activity.

The antimicrobial agents can be introduced into polymer microparticles. The co-precipitation of $CaCO_3$ and silver nanoparticles (SNPs) in the presence of poly(sodium 4-styrenesulfonate) leads to a system that enables sustained release of biocide [26]. Microbiological tests confirmed the effectiveness of these microparticles as an antibacterial agent. This designed material can be stored as a dry powder and subsequently re-suspended in water without the risk of losing its antimicrobial activity.

Plasma is widely used as a tool for polymer functionalization with biocide agents. SNPs-based antibacterial coatings can protect eukaryotic cells from SNPs-related toxic effects, while preserving antibacterial efficiency [27]. A system of SNPs containing n-heptylamine (HA) polymer matrix was deposited by plasma polymerization and covered by a second HA layer. Even so, the antibacterial activity is maintained to planktonic bacteria living in the near surroundings of the material. The SNPs-based materials also revealed antibacterial effect on adhered bacteria [28, 29]. Their number was significantly reduced compared to pure HA plasma polymer and the physiology of the bacteria was affected. The number of adhered bacteria is directly diminished with thickness of the second HA layer.

5. *In Vivo* and *In vitro* activity of antibacterial substances

Bacterial agents can cause both superficial and serious systemic diseases, generating infections anywhere, including in hospitals. Infections involve the formation of *in vitro* or *in vivo* bio-clusters on implanted devices, such as catheters or prosthetic heart valves. These bacterial agents formed *in vitro* on different bio-materials consist of micro-colonies which are resistant to a range of antibacterial agents, through several mechanisms of resistance [30, 31]. Microorganisms can be organized as biofilms, including pathogens, thus offering a means to protect themselves against antimicrobial agents. Several mechanisms have been proposed to explain this phenomenon of resistance within biofilms, such as:

- delayed penetration of the antimicrobial into the biofilm extracellular matrix;
- slowing of growth rate of organisms within the biofilm
- physiologic changes brought about by interaction of the organisms with a surface.

Implications of biofilm formation are that alternative control strategies must be devised both for testing the susceptibility of the organisms within the biofilm and for treating the established biofilm to alter its structure. A number of testing protocols have been developed. The effective treatment strategies include antimicrobials or other agents that can penetrate and kill the biofilm organisms, or treatments that can disrupt or target specific components of the biofilm matrix [32].

Recent studies on bacterial and fungal species suggest that extensive and striking interactions occur between the prokaryotic and eukaryotic cells [33]. Also, their possible mechanisms of resistance vary with the nature of the administered antimicrobial agent, are not fully understood, and are grouped in literature taking into account [34] the following parameters:

- Restricted penetration of drugs through the micro-colonies
- Phenotypic changes resulting from a decreased growth rate or nutrient limitation
- Nature of resistance genes induced by contact with a surface
- Number of 'per-sister' cells considered responsible for resistance

The methods of selection of drugs to be considerate in case of combined devices are provided by Venn diagram---a diagram (Figure 5) that shows all possible logical relations between finite collections of different sets, including the pharmaceutical device (pharmacokinetics, pharmacodynamics, biopharmaceutics, therapeutic dose), medical device (type and class of device, manufacturing process, testing requirements), and combination device perspective (local drug effects, controlled release combined manufactured methods, business drivers, clinical concerns) [33].

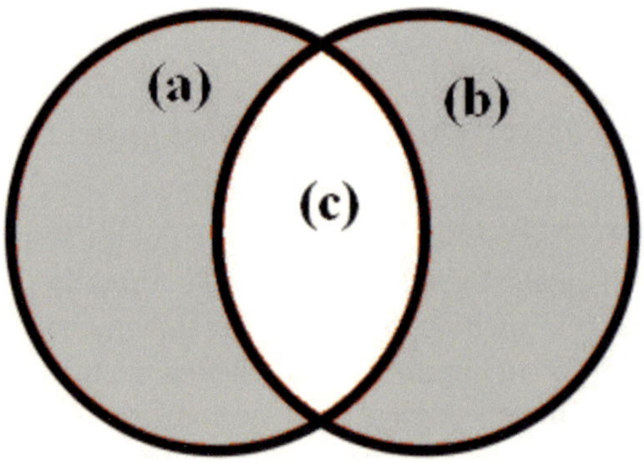

Figure 5. The Venn diagram for perspective of devices and combined devices: (a) pharmaceutical device; (b) medical device; and (c) combination device

The considerable interest exists in combination devices that include the type of peripheral stents, orthopedics, indwelling catheters, dental implants, surgical meshes, wound dressings, ophthalmic implants, sutures, and even artificial organs [35, 36]. The physicochemical properties of the drugs used in combination devices, as well as their location in vivo or in vitro, include the knowledge of their antibacterial activity.

Table 1 presents the beneficial effects of treatment with antimicrobial agents against various types of bacteria, associated as biofilms.

However, besides the beneficial treatments, there are some secondary effects produced by antimicrobial drugs. The fluoroquinolone class of antibacterial drugs that determine adverse events include central nervous system toxicity, phototoxicity, and in some cases electrocardiographic changes. Some side-effects of the quinolones are class effects, and cannot be modulated by molecular variation. These include gastrointestinal irritation and arthropathy.

Tested bacteria	Antibacterial drug	
Escherichia coli	Cefazolin, ciprofloxacin, clindamycin, gentamicin, oxacillin, penicillin, vancomycin	[37]
Escherichia coli	Latamoxef	[38]
Pseudomonas aeruginosa	Cefazolin, ciprofloxacin, clindamycin, gentamicin, oxacillin, penicillin, vancomycin	[37]
Pseudomonas aeruginosa	Cefuroxime, piperacillin, tobramycin, vancomycin	[39]
Staphylococus aureus	Cefazolin, ciprofloxacin, clindamycin, gentamicin, oxacillin, penicillin, vancomycin	[37]
Staphylococus aureus	Cefazolin, cefuzonam, cephalexin, gentamicin, ofloxacin, tosufloxacin	[40]
Staphylococus aureus	Cefazolin, cefuroxime, bioluminescence ciprofloxacin, erythromycin, gentamicin, novobiocin, penicillin G, phosphomycin, rifampin, tobramycin, vancomycin	[41]
Staphylococus aureus	Fleroxacin, gentamicin, oxacillin, vancomycin	[42]
Staphylococus aureus	Cefuroxime	[39]
Staphylococus aureus	Vancomycin, teicoplanin	[43]
Staphylococus epidermidis	Ciprofloxacin, quinupristin/dalfopristin Vancomycin	[44]
Staphylococus. epidermidis	Ciprofloxacin	[45]
Staphylococus epidermidis	Cefuroxime, piperacillin, tobramycin, vancomycin	[39]
Staphylococus epidermidis	Amikacin, levofloxacin, rifampin, teicoplanin	[46]
Streptococcus pneumoniae	Vancomycin, teicoplanin	[43]

Table 1. Response to antibiotics of different bacteria associated as biofilms

Moreover, gastrointestinal prokinetics, such as metoclopramide, cisapride and levosulpiride, are widely used for the management of functional gut disorders. Recent investigations revealed that cisapride (a partial 5-HT4 receptor agonist) can generate dose-dependent cardiac adverse effects, including lengthening of the electrocardiographic QT interval, syncopal episodes, and ventricular dysrhythmias.

Determination of the minimum inhibitory concentration, based on the activities of antibiotics against planktonic bacteria, is the standard assay for antibiotic susceptibility testing. In this context, the Calgary Biofilm Device is well recognized as a technology for the rapid and reproducible assay of biofilm susceptibilities to antibiotics, for the rational selection of antibiotics effective against microbial biofilms, and for the finding of new effective antibiotic compounds [8]. On the other hand, the antibiotic tolerance is defined as the ability of bacteria to survive but not grow in the presence of antibiotics. It is known that adherent bacteria on solid surfaces already have tolerance to antibiotics and depend essentially on the different stress conditions on antibiotic tolerance [47]. The rise in antibiotic resistance among pathogenic bacteria and the declining rate of novel drug discovery motivate recent studies to find new classes of antibacterial agents and novel drugs, in order to maintain the ability to treat infectious diseases---especially those caused by multidrug-resistant organisms [48]. Research concerning the activity and design of cationic antimicrobial peptides and their mimics has produced several antimicrobial compounds with good antibacterial activity and elucidated trends of increasing activity and specificity. Applications are numerous, including antimicrobial surfaces [49] and conjugates in targeted therapy [50].

The interest in cationic antimicrobial peptides opens new perspectives in antimicrobial drug design. The Hunter-killer peptides represent a novel class of targeted peptides that have demonstrated remarkable efficacy in several basic proof-of-principle paradigms including therapeutics for cancer [51], arthritis [52], prostate reduction [53], and obesity [54]. There are also reported new hunter-killer "nanostructures/nanospheres" and second-generation Hunter-killer peptides derivatives, which are protected from proteolytic degradation and adjust their "modulation of the absorption, distribution, metabolism, and excretion" properties [55]. This technology uses similar way to encapsulate anticancer proteins, such as the small globular proteins. Development and evaluation of the next generation of Hunter-killer peptides with improved modulation of the absorption, distribution, metabolism, and excretion properties are studies currently underway.

Host-defense peptides are present components of the innate immune system across all organisms. These molecules have been widely studied for their activities, such as antimicrobial, antitumor, mitogenic, and chemical signaling properties. It is known that oligo-acyl-lysyls are synthetic mimics of host-defense peptides known to exert antibacterial activity both in cultures and in animal models of disease [56]. Data obtained with representative bacteria, including the Gram-negative bacterium *Escherichia coli* and the Gram-positive bacteria *Listeria monocytogenes* and *Staphylococcus aureus*, shows that the oligo-acyl-lysyls potency is affected by pH changes and subsides essentially throughout a wide range of salt concentrations and temperature, whereas antistaphyloccocal activity is vulnerable. Also, in biomedical strategy concerning host-defense peptides, several short synthetic oligomers such as methacrylate, arylamide foldamers, and oligo-acyl-lysyls have attracted particular attention due to their lower cost and rapid structural optimization capabilities [57]. Although a number of compounds that demonstrate broad-spectrum antimicrobial activities *in vitro* have been identified, robust/safe *in vivo* activity has been a great challenge for most published peptidomimetics [58]. As a result of the appearance of multidrug-resistant bacteria, antimicrobial peptides have emerged as one of the leading prospects for drug development. Antimicrobial peptides are retained in a wide range of organisms as a defense mechanism against a broad array of microbial targets. These peptides vary in size, sequence, and efficacy, allowing a good interaction with the charged bacterial membrane [59]. In this context, to mimic the amphiphilic nature of antimicrobial peptides, arylamide foldamers were prepared, that demonstrated bactericidal activity against both Gram-negative and Gram-positive strains, without many of the drawbacks of natural antimicrobial peptides [60].

http://dx.doi.org/10.5772/60755

The emergence and spread of antibiotic resistance represent an alarming concern in clinical practice. From this reason, the antimicrobial agents are used to cover materials and medical devices as a prophylaxis to prevent bacteria from growing or for therapeutic uses. A range of silver-coated or impregnated dressings are commercially available for use. The antibacterial activities of silver-coated/impregnated dressings were compared against common burn-wound pathogens, namely *Staphylococcus aureus, Enterococcus faecalis, Pseudomonas aeruginosa, Escherichia coli, Enterobacter cloacae, Proteus vulgaris, Acinetobacter baumannii.* The rapidity and extent of killing of these pathogens evaluated under *in vitro* conditions shows that silver-impregnated dressings exert bactericidal activity, particularly against Gram-negative bacteria, including *Enterobacter* species, *Proteus* species, and *Escherichia coli.* Therefore, the incorporation of silver for dressings or as coating on medical products plays an important role in the domain of antimicrobial agents [61].

On the other hand, it is known that infection is the most common cause of biomaterial implant failure in modern medicine [62]. Adhesion and subsequent surface growth of bacteria on biomedical implants and devices cause the formation of a biofilm, in which the so-called "glycocalyx" embeds the infecting bacteria offering protection against the host immune system and antibiotic treatment. Gram-positive *Staphylococcus aureus* and *Staphylococcus epidermidis* are the predominant infecting organisms, followed by Gram-negative bacilli like *Escherichia coli* and *Pseudomonas aeruginosa.* A possible approach to prevent biomaterial-centered infections is to render the biomaterial surface antimicrobial properties by functionalization with, e.g., quaternary ammonium groups, which are widely known as disinfectants. Quaternary ammonium-functionalized surfaces have a high positive surface charge, and thus exert a strong adhesive force on negatively charged bacteria which are proposed to inhibit surface growth of bacteria. The main mechanisms of action of antibacterial drugs (Figure 6) can be classified as follows:

- Inhibition of cell wall synthesis (amoxicillin, cefalexin, oxacilin)
- Inhibition of protein synthesis (chloramphenicol, clarithromycin, erythromycin)
- Inhibition of nucleic acid synthesis (ciprofloxacin, norfloxacin, novobiocin)
- Inhibition of metabolic pathways (sulphanilamide, trimethoprim)
- Interference with cell membrane integrity (cerulenin, triclosan)

Several *in vitro* and *in vivo* studies show that methicillin-resistant *Staphylococcus aureus* (MRSA) remains a leading cause of bacterial infections worldwide, ranging from minor skin and soft tissue infections to more severe conditions such as bacteremia and infective endocarditis [63]. The molecules currently under pre-clinical and clinical investigation that are active against MRSA, with special emphasis on their mechanism of action are grouped as follows:

- Molecules acting on peptidoglycan biosynthesis and the cell membrane (lipopeptides, lipoglycopeptides, cell membrane inhibitors)
- Protein synthesis inhibitors (oxazolidinones, aminomethylcyclines, aminoglycosides, peptide deformylase inhibitors)

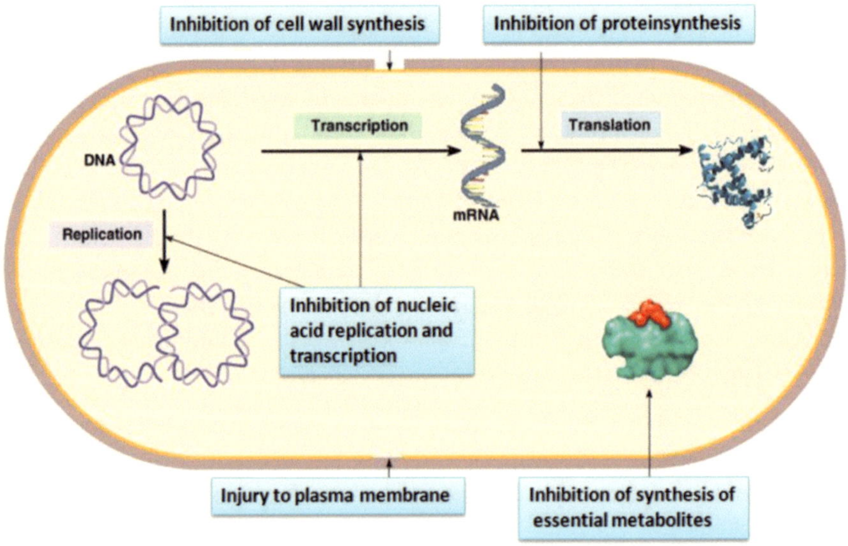

Figure 6. The main action mechanisms of antibacterial drugs

- DNA synthesis inhibitors (fluoroquinolones, dihydrofolate reductase inhibitors)
- Fatty acid synthesis inhibitors

As can be seen here, drug discovery and development against MRSA is a highly active field. The wide-ranging clinical spectrum of infections is mirrored by the discovery of chemical classes active against it [63]. Literature offers the opportunity to obtain a new drug with antibacterial, antifungal, antiviral, and antiparasitic potential from natural products by extraction process. Cos et al. [64] presents a scheme of testing organisms for antibacterial, antifungal, antiviral, and antiparasitic screening *in vitro*. Irrespective of the adopted plant collection strategy, a critical step is the processing of the plant material that will be used in the process of screens. Infections caused by different species continue to increase in frequency and severity [65]. The number of enzymes and the number of organisms that exhibit cross-resistance to some classes of antimicrobials is growing, generating an increase of researches in antibacterial substances domain.

6. Conclusion and future perspectives

The treatment of infections caused by bacteria remains an actual problem that still raises problems and maintains a vivid interest of both scientists and pharmaceutical companies for finding new and innovative solutions. These health issues should be approached on multiple levels, starting from synthesis, design, and the mechanisms of action. The research directed towards the preparation of new antibacterial compounds must be based on deeper understanding of the resistance mechanisms. More promising antibacterial drugs with novel mechanisms of action should be developed and new types of targets must emerge. There is a great need for enhancing the precision of targeting the pathogens and limit the misuse of antimicrobials and other practices that accelerate the emergence of novel resistance mechanisms. So, specific microbial target enzymes will continue to attract attention for novel antimicrobial discovery. A starting point is given by peptide deformylase, but its unstable character delays its utilization on industrial level. Advances in deciphering the genome of a several microbes will further help the discovery of agents against them by providing a wider selection of potential targets.

Another emerging trend for the future is the increasing correlation between infections and other diseases. For example, infection with *Chlamydia pneumoniae* is a determining factor in the pathogenesis of atherosclerosis. Administration of specific drugs was found to be protective against atherosclerosis complications, thus reducing the disease progression in as yet unspecified ways. This type of significant correlation will be taken into increasing account by antibacterial drug producers in the future, as the repercussions of infection, and therefore treatment, expand beyond the microbe itself.

On the other hand, although there is a major progress on designing scientifically sound and feasible clinical trials, more efforts must be made for making new therapies available to meet patient needs. On the other hand, novel strategies, like targeting host infection response pathways or anti-infective antibodies, offer an insight into the anti-infective drug discovery pipeline of the future.

Acknowledgements

This work was financially supported from PNII-ID-PCE-2011-3-0937 Project No. 302/5.10.2011.

Author details

Andreea Irina Barzic and Silvia Ioan*

*Address all correspondence to: ioan_silvia@yahoo.com

Department of Physical Chemistry of Polymers, "Petru Poni" Institute of Macromolecular Chemistry, Iasi, Romania

References

[1] Bobbarala V, Vadlapudi V. Abrus precatorius l. seed extracts antimicrobial properties against clinically important bacteria. Int J Pharm Tech Res. 2009;1:1115-1118.

[2] Jenkins SG, Farrell D J. Increase in pneumococcus macrolide resistance. Emerg Infect Dis. 2009;15:1260-1264. DOI: 10.3201/eid1508.081187

[3] Rossi F, García P, Ronzon B, Curcio D, Dowzicky MJ. Rates of antimicrobial resistance in Latin America (2004-2007) and in vitro activity of the glycylcycline tigecycline and of other antibiotics. Braz J Infect Dis. 2008;12:405-415. DOI: 10.1590/S1413-86702008000500012

[4] Czyż DM, Potluri L-P, Jain-Gupta N, et al. Host-directed antimicrobial drugs with broad-spectrum efficacy against intracellular bacterial pathogens. mBio. 2014;5:e01534-14. DOI: 10.1128/mBio.01534-14

[5] Devasahayam G, Scheld WM, Hoffman PS. Newer antibacterial drugs for a new century. Expert Opin Investig Drugs. 2010;19:215-234. DOI: 10.1517/13543780903505092

[6] Abbanat D, Morrow B, Bush K. New agents in development for the treatment of bacterial infections. Curr Opin Pharmacol. 2008;8:582-592. DOI: 10.1016/j.coph.2008.08.001

[7] Fiege H, Voges HW, Hamamoto T, et al. "Phenol Derivatives." In: Ullmann's Encyclopedia of Industrial Chemistry. Wiley, 2002; DOI: 10.1002/14356007.a19_313

[8] Wright PM, Seiple IB, Myers AG. The evolving role of chemical synthesis in antibacterial drug discovery. Angew Chem Int Ed Engl. 2014;53:8840-8869. DOI: 10.1002/anie.201310843

[9] Naeem A, Haque S, Khan RH. Purification and characterization of a novel beta-D-galactosides-specific lectin from Clitoria ternatea. Protein J. 2007;26:403-413.

[10] Medeiros DS, Medeiros TL, Ribeiro JK, et al. A lactose specific lectin from the sponge Cinachyrella apion: purification, characterization, N-terminal sequences alignment and agglutinating activity on Leishmania promastigotes. Comp Biochem Physiol B. 2010;155:211-216. DOI: 10.1016/j.cbpb.2009.10.016

[11] Estebanez A, Pascual R, Gil V, et al. Fosfomycin in a single dose versus a 7-day course of amoxicillin–clavulanate for the treatment of asymptomatic bacteriuria during pregnancy. Eur J Clin Microbiol Infect Dis. 2009;28:1457-1464. DOI: 10.1007/s10096-009-0805-6

[12] Rogers T, Birnbaum J. Biosynthesis of Fosfomycin by Streptomyces fradiae. Antimicrobial Agents Chemother. 1974;5:121-132.

[13] Marocco CP, Davis EV, Finnell JE, et al. Asymmetric synthesis of (−)-fosfomycin and its trans-(1S,2S)-diastereomer using a biocatalytic reduction as the key step. Tetrahedron: Asymmetry. 2011;22:1784-1789. DOI: 10.1016/j.tetasy.2011.10.009

[14] Shih DH, Baker F, Cama L, Christensen BG. Synthetic Carbapenem Antibiotics. I. 1-β-Methylcarbapenem. Heterocycles. 1984;21:29-40. DOI: 10.3987/S-1984-01-0029

[15] Sneader W. Drug Discovery: A History. ed. Chichester: Wiley, 2005; p. 469. DOI: 10.1002/0470015535

[16] Hitchings GH, Elion GB, Van derWerff H, Falco EA. Pyrimidine derivatives as antagonists of pteroylglutamic acid. J Biol Chem. 1948;174:765-766.

[17] Ippolito JA, Kanyo Z F, Wang D, et al. Crystal structure of the oxazolidinone antibiotic linezolid bound to the 50S ribosomal subunit. J Med Chem. 2008;51:3353-3356. DOI: 10.1021/jm800379d

[18] Siedenbiedel F, Tiller JC. Antimicrobial polymers in solution and on surfaces: Overview and functional principles. Polymers. 2012;4:46-71. DOI: 10.3390/polym4010046

[19] Timofeeva L, Kleshcheva N. Antimicrobial polymers: Mechanism of action, factors of activity, and applications. Appl Microbiol Biotechnol. 2011;89:475-492. DOI: 10.1007/s00253-010-2920-9

[20] Dizman B, Elasri MO, Mathias LJ. Synthesis, characterization, and antibacterial activities of novel methacrylate polymers containing norfloxacin. Biomacromolecules. 2005;6:514-520.

[21] Kawabata N, Nishiguchi M. Antibacterial activity of soluble pyridinium-type polymers. Appl Environ Microbiol. 1988;54:2532-2535.

[22] Kanazawa A, Ikeda T, Endo T. Polymeric phosphonium salts as a novel class of cationic biocides IV synthesis and antibacterial activity of polymers with phosphonium salts in the main chain. J Polym Sci Part A. 1993;31:3031-3038. DOI: 10.1002/pola.1993.080311219

[23] Kanazawa A, Ikeda T, Endo T. Antibacterial activity of polymeric sulfonium salts. J Polym Sci Part A. 1993;31:2873-2876. DOI: 10.1002/pola.1993.080311126

[24] Ruszczak Z, Friess W. Collagen as a carrier for on-site delivery of antibacterial drugs. Adv Drug Deliv. Rev. 2003;55:1679-1698. DOI: 10.1016/j.addr.2003.08.007

[25] Kugel A, Chisholm B, Ebert S, et al. Antimicrobial polysiloxane polymers and coatings containing pendant levofloxacin. Polym Chem. 2010;1:442-452. DOI: 10.1039/b9py00309f

[26] Długosz M, Bulwan M, Kania G, Nowakowska M, Zapotoczny S. Hybrid calcium carbonate/polymer microparticles containing silver nanoparticles as antibacterial agents. J Nanopart Res. 2012;14:1313-1320. DOI:10.1007/s11051-012-1313-7

[27] Ploux L, Mateescu M, Anselme K, Vasilev K. Antibacterial properties of silver-loaded plasma polymer coatings. J Nanomater. 2012;2012:1-9. DOI: 10.1155/2012/674145

[28] Necula AM, Dunca S, Stoica I, et al. Morphological properties and antibacterial activity of nano-silver-containing cellulose acetate phthalate films. Int J Polym Anal Charact. 2010;15:341-350. DOI: 10.1080/1023666X.2010.500524

[29] Ioan S, Filimon A. Biocompatibility and antimicrobial activity of some quaternized polysulfones. In: Biochemistry, Genetics and Molecular Biology: A Search for Antibacterial Agents. ed. Croatia: InTech; 2012; p. 249-274. DOI: 10.5772/33053

[30] Mah TFC, O'Toole GA. Mechanisms of biofilm resistance to antimicrobial agents. Trends Microbiol. 2001;9:34-39.

[31] Douglas LJ. Candida biofilms and their role in infection. Trends Microbiol. 2003;11:30-36.

[32] Donland RM. Role of biofilms in antimicrobial resistance. ASAIO J. 2000;46:S47-S52.

[33] Hupcey MAZ, Ekins S. Improving the drug selection and development process for combination devices. Drug Discov. Today. 2007;12:844-852.

[34] [34]Lewis K. Riddle of biofilm resistance. Antimicrob Agents Chemother. 2001;45:999-1007.

[35] Wu P, Grainger DW. Drug/device combinations for local drug therapies and infection prophylaxis. Biomaterials. 2006;27:2450-2467.

[36] Phaneuf MD, Bide JM, Hannel SL, et al. Development of an infection-resistant, bioactive wound dressing surface. J Biomed Mater Res Part A. 2005;74:666-676.

[37] Ceri H, Olson ME, Stremick C, et al. The Calgary biofilm device: New technology for rapid determination of antibiotic susceptibilities of bacterial biofilms. J Clin Microbiol. 1999;37:1771-1776.

[38] Jouenne T, Tresse O, Junter GA. Agar-entrapped bacteria as an in vitro model of biofilms and their susceptibility to antibiotics. FEMS Microbiol Lett. 1994;119:237-242.

[39] Domingue G, Ellis B, Dasgupta M, Costerton JW. Testing antimicrobial susceptibilities of adherent bacteria by a method that incorporates guidelines of the National Committee for Clinical Laboratory Standards. J Clin Microbiol. 1994;32:2564-2568.

[40] Miyake Y, Fujiwara S, Usui T, Suginaka H. Simple method for measuring the antibiotic concentration required to kill adherent bacteria. Chemotherapy. 1992;38:286-290.

[41] Amorena B, Gracia E, Monzón M, et al. Antibiotic susceptibility assay for Staphylococcus aureus in biofilms developed *in vitro*. J Antimicrob Chemother. 1999;44:43-55.

[42] Eng RHK, Hsieh A, Smith SM. Antibiotic killing of bacteria: Comparison of bacteria on surfaces and in liquid, growing and nongrowing. Chemotherapy. 1995;41:113-120.

[43] Knudes J, Fuursted K, Raber S, Espersen F, Frimodt-Moller N. Pharmacodynamics of glycopeptides in the mouse peritonitis model of Streptococcus pneumoniae or Staphylococcus aureus infection. Antimicrob Agents Chemother. 2000;44:1247-1254.

[44] Hamilton-Miller JMT, Shah S. Activity of quinupristin/dalfopristin against Staphylococcus epidermidis in biofilms: A comparison with ciprofloxacin. J Antimicrob Chemother (Suppl A). 1997;39:103-108.

[45] Duguid IG, Evans E, Brown MRW, Gilbert P. Growth-rate-independent killing by ciprofloxacin of biofilm-derived Staphylococcus epidermidis: Evidence for cell-cycle dependency. J Antimicrob Chemother. 1992;30:791-802.

[46] Schwank S, Rajacic Z, Zimmerli W, Blaser J. Impact of bacterial biofilm formation on in vitro and in vivo activities of antibiotics. Antimicrob Agents Chemother. 1998;42:895-898.

[47] Murakami K, Ono T, Viducic D, et al. Role for rpoS gene of Pseudomonas aeruginosa in antibiotic tolerance. FEMS Microbiol Lett. 2005;242:161-167.

[48] Findlay B, Zhanel GG, Schweizer F. Cationic amphiphiles, a new generation of antimicrobials inspired by the natural antimicrobial peptide scaffold. Antimicrob Agents Chemother. 2010;54:4049-4058.

[49] Madkour, AE, Dabkowski JM, Nusslein K, Tew GN. Fast disinfecting antimicrobial surfaces. Langmuir. 2009;25:1060-1067. DOI: 10.1021/la802953v

[50] Ellerby HM, Bredesen DE, Fujimura S, John V. Hunterkiller peptide (HKP) for targeted therapy. J Med Chem. 2008;51:5887-5892. DOI: 10.1021/jm800495u

[51] Ellerby HM, Arap W, Ellerby LM, et al. Anti-cancer activity of targeted pro-apoptotic peptides. Nat Med. 1999;5:1032-1038. DOI: 10.1038/12469

[52] Gerlag DM, Borges E, Tak PP, et al. Suppression of murine collagen-induced arthritis by targeted apoptosis of synovial neovasculature. Arthritis Res. 2001;3:357-361.

[53] Arap W, Haedicke W, Bernasconi M, et al. Targeting the prostate for destruction through a vascular address. Proc Natl Acad Sci U S A. 2002;99:1527-1531. DOI: 10.1073/pnas.241655998

[54] Kolonin MG, Saha PK, Chan L, Pasqualini R, Arap W. Reversal of obesity by targeted ablation of adipose tissue. Nat Med. 2004;10:625-632.

[55] Michael Ellerby HM, Bredesen DE, Fujimura S, John V. Hunter-Killer Peptide (HKP) for targeted therapy. J Medicinal Chem. 2008;51:5887-5892. DOI: 10.1021/jm800495u

[56] Goldfeder Y, Zaknoon F, Mor A. Experimental conditions that enhance potency of an antibacterial oligo-acyl-lysyl. Antimicrob Agents Chemother. 2010;54:2590-2595. DOI: 10.1128/AAC.01656-09

[57] Mor A. Chemical mimics with systemic efficacy. In: Antimicrobial Peptides: Discovery, Design and Novel Therapeutic Strategies. Wallingford: CABI Publishing; 2010; p. 100-115. DOI: 10.1079/9781845936570.0100

[58] Zaknoon F, Goldberg K, Sarig H, et al. Antibacterial properties of an oligo-acyl-lysyl hexamer targeting gram-negative species. Antimicrob Agents Chemother. 2012;56:4827-4832. DOI: 10.1128/AAC.00511-12

[59] Glukhov E, Burrows LL, Deber CM. Membrane interactions of designed cationic antimicrobial peptides: The two thresholds. Biopolymers. 2008;89:360-371. DOI: 10.1002/bip.20917

[60] Mensa B, Kim YH, Choi S, et al. Antibacterial mechanism of action of arylamide foldamers. Antimicrob Agents Chemother. 2011;55:5043-5053. DOI: 10.1128/AAC.05009-11.

[61] Ip M, Lui SL, Poo VCM, Lung I, Burd A. Antimicrobial activities of silver dressings: An in vitro comparison. J Med Microbiol. 2006;55:59-63.

[62] Gottenbos B, van der Mei HC, Klatter F, Nieuwenhuis P, Busscher HJ. *In vitro* and *in vivo* antimicrobial activity of covalently coupled quaternary ammonium silane coatings on silicone rubber. Biomaterials. 2002;23:1417-1423.

[63] Kumar K, Chopra S. New drugs for methicillin-resistant Staphylococcus aureus: An update. J Antimicrob Chemother. 2013;68:1465-1470. DOI: 10.1093/jac/dkt045

[64] Cos P, Vlietinck AJ, Vanden Berghe DV, Maesa L. Anti-infective potential of natural products: How to develop a stronger in vitro 'proof-of-concept.' J Ethnopharm. 2006;106:290-302. DOI: 10.1016/j.jep.2006.04.003

[65] Nemeth J, Oesch G, Kuster SP. Bacteriostatic versus bactericidal antibiotics for patients with serious bacterial infections: Systematic review and meta-analysis. J Antimicrob Chemother. 2015;70:382-395.

Chapter 2

Perception and Resistance Mechanism of some Metal-drug Complexes and Their Roles as Antibacterial

Joshua A. Obaleye, Nzikahyel Simon, Olufunso O. Abosede, Mercy O. Bamigboye, Abiodun A. Ajibola, Uche B. Eke and Elizabeth A. Balogun

Additional information is available at the end of the chapter

http://dx.doi.org/10.5772/61033

Abstract

Metal-based drugs have undergone much development and application for therapeutic and diagnostic purposes for many decades since the huge success of cisplatin and other successful metal-drug complexes in the clinical stages. Furthermore, this metal-based drug has come up with a lot of signs of resistance and side-effects in their uses. This review points to some of the resistance natures and mechanisms of previously synthesized complexes in the field of chemistry.

Keywords: metal-drug complexes, antibacterial, mechanism, therapeutics, properties, resistance

1. Introduction

Anti-bacterial are agents that disturb and combat the growth and reproduction of bacteria. They are known as agents used to disinfect surfaces and eliminate potentially harmful bacteria. Some antibacterial agents are contraindicated while some required dosage modification in patients who have renal insufficiency. The use of metal complexes as antibacterial/chemotherapeutic agents against some ailments is a very attractive potential. Some metal complexes including mixed ligand metal complexes have been prepared in our laboratory and that of others. Their effectiveness as antibacterial agents has been revealed. Different synthetic procedures were utilized.

Though development of metallo-pharmaceuticals is met with limitations because of the perception that metals (especially when regarded as heavy metals) are toxic and the relative limited expertise of most pharmaceutical companies in Inorganic Chemistry, metals and their compounds are essential to many species of plants and animals. Metal complexes may be useful as research probes of biological function, as intermediary lead compounds in the development of non-metal-containing therapeutics, and as potential diagnostic and therapeutic agents. The unique properties of metal complexes,(e. g., hydrolytic and redox activity, valency, geometry, magnetic, spectroscopic, photo-physical, and radiochemical properties) can be used to measure and/or alter cellular functions. In the recent past, polypyridyl metal complexes are also being tested as chemotherapeutic agents following the first success of cisplatin and the need to discover new drugs to combat the problem of resistance to existing drugs [1-8].

The importance of metal in medicine has been in existence for many years and researchers have explored their uses and advantages to human health, animals and the environment. Some of these metals are content of our day-to-day diets and in varying quantities.

Many researchers have come up with the importance of metals in known drugs or synthesized drugs. Transition metals are involved majorly in the formation of complexes by coordinating with the ligands (i. e. the drugs).

Humans need several metal ions for many vital and important functions in the body in which the lack of some of these metal ions can lead to malfunctioning of the body and development of diseases. Iron deficiency can lead to pernicious anemia while copper deficiency in infants can cause lack of accurate function of the heart.

Medicinal bioinorganic chemistry considers, from a molecular level point of view, how to understand and recognize different diseases that originate from the deficiency of essential metal ions functionality in the body of a living system. This also includes ways of providing solution to these problems. Introduction of heavy metal ions (e. g., Pb and Hg) can be detrimental to living systems [9].

The involvement of the metal ions in most of these potent synthesized complexes has increased their biological activities. In most cases the acceleration of the action of many drugs is mainly caused by metal ion chelation. Therefore many metals are involved in enhancing the efficacy in antimalarial, antitumor and anticancer therapy [10-13].

Drug resistance refers to a situation in which the drugs that usually destroy the bacteria can no longer perform its duty. It implies that the patient can no longer be effectively treated against the bacteria.

Therefore, people become sick for a long time and if the epidemics are extended without a possible solution it results in more people being at risk of becoming infected.

Antimicrobial resistance is the ability of a microorganism to survive at a given concentration of anantimicrobial agent at which the normal population of the microorganism would be killed.

2. Resistance of some metal-drug complexes of antimalarial

2.1. Resistance to anti-malarials

Resistance to antimalarials could be defined as the tendency by which the parasite is able to thrive and even reproduce itself in the presence of accurate dosage of malaria drug [14].

In 2006, the World Health Organisation (WHO) stated that, resistance has arisen to all classes of anti-malarials except the artemisinins. This has increased the malaria burden globally and is a most important threat to malaria control. Extensive and indiscriminate uses of antimalarial drugs impose a strong selective stress on *Plasmodium falciparum* and other malaria parasites to acquire higher resistance levels. This can be prevented at its onset or mellowed down significantly, through combination therapies of the anti-malarial drugs with differing modes of actions thereby achieving maximum cure rates by strict adherence to proper drug prescriptions [13].

The data acquired can be of assistance in treatment choices and forecasts concerning future resistance patterns. The most difficult with drug resistance arises from *P. falciparum*. Resistance due to *P. falciparum* is of special interest since the huge burden of disease arises from this class, as well as its deadly potential, the tendency for epidemics, and the cost implication of replacement with candidate drugs in places with well-known drug resistance. Chloroquine resistance does occur in *P. vivax*, particularly in Western Oceania. However, there is very scanty information on resistance in *P. ovale* and *P. malariae* [14].

Malaria is a deadly disease that affect both children and adult and is mostly caused by the protozoan parasite *Plasmodium*, and is transmitted by an Anopheline mosquito vector [15]. The five Plasmodia species affecting humans are *Plasmodium falciparum, Plasmodium vivax, Plasmodium ovale, Plasmodium malariae,* and *Plasmodium knowlesi. Plasmodium falciparum* is a common species commonly affecting the population and therefore its resistance to many drugs. Today, the available therapeutic drugs for malaria are limited; new anti-malarial drugs, preferably with new structures and/or modes of action, are urgently needed [16, 17].

The emergence of resistance in *Plasmodium* depends on parasite mutation rate and their total parasite load. Treatment response and drug selection strength also contributed to these factors.

Increase in the rates of mutation enhances the speed of resistance emergence which subsequently leads to harmful mutations [17].

3. Some metal-drug complexes resistance and their mechanism

3.1. Metal complexes of antimalarial drugs

Metal–drug synergism has been exploited to obtain effective antimalarial metal agents [18-20].

The use of chloroquine (CQ) as a major reference drug of all antimalarial drugs has enabled many scientists to develop more potent drugs in combating malaria. Resistance against CQ is now prominent. The incorporation of metals into CQ and similar drugs has been yielding more positive results with little or no toxicity. Some examples of synthesized metal- drug complexes including their various resistances are also cited in the table below:

For Ruthenium and Rhodium complexes of chloroquine:

(A)

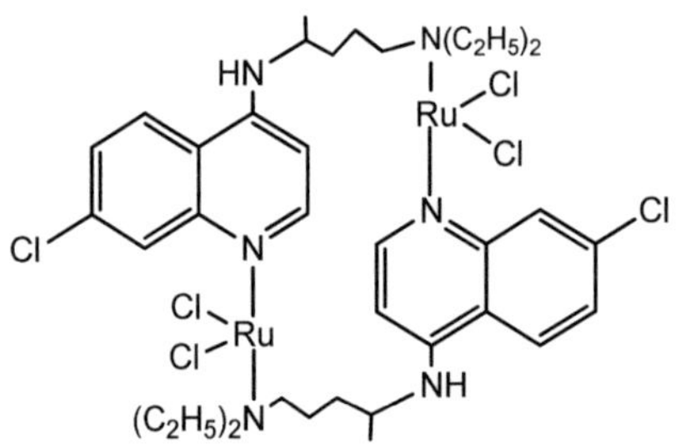

Ru-chloroquine

$[RuCQCl_2]_2$

(B)

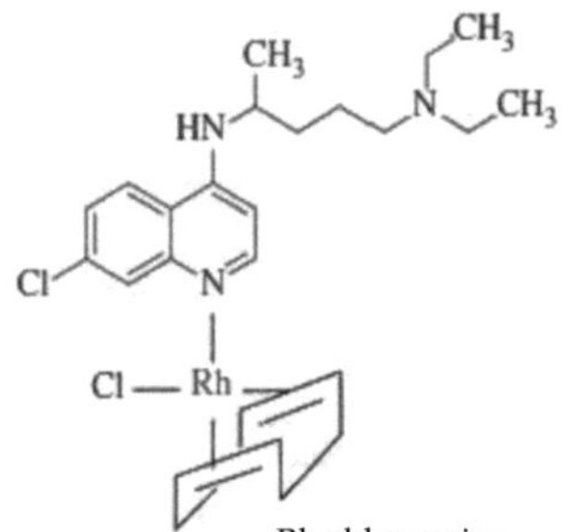

Rh-chloroquine

RhCl(COD)CQ

Compound	CQ-Sensitive strains	CQ-Resistance strains	Reference
A	*P. berghei*	FcB1, FcB2	[21]
B	Reduction of parasitemia by 73%	FcB1	[21]

Where (COD: 1,5-Cyclooctadiene), Ru- Ruthenium, Rh= Rhenium,

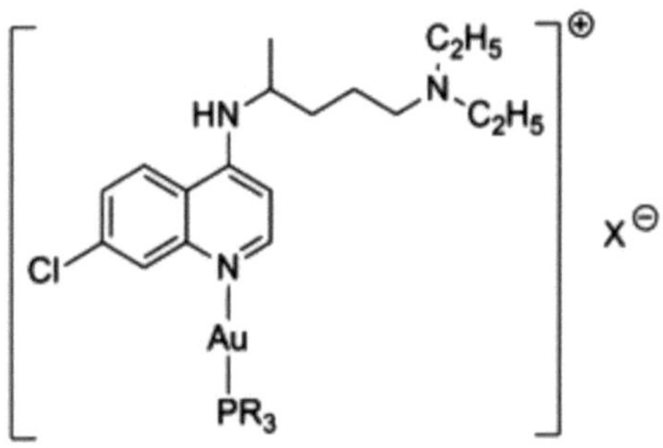

1. **R = CH_3, X= PF_6 (Au-CQ)**
2. **R = C_6H_5, X = PF_6**
3. **R = C_6H_5, X = NO_3**
4. **R = C_2H_5, X = PF_6**

Compound	CQ-Sensitive strains of P. berghei	CQ-Resistance strains of P. falciparum	Reference
1. $[Au(PMe_3)(CQ)]PF_6]$	F32	W2, K1, FcB1	[23]
2. $[Au(PPh_3)(CQ)]PF_6$	F32	FcB1, FcB2	[22]
3. $[Au(PPh_3)(CQ)]NO_3$	F32	W2, K1, FcB1	[23]
4. $[Au(PEt_3)(CQ)]PF_6$	F32	W2, K1, FcB1	[22]

From the conclusion that was drawn from the mechanism of $[Au(PPh_3)(CQ)]PF_6$ and its antimalarial action, $[Au(PPh_3)(CQ)]PF_6$ has high propensity to haem than chloroquine diphosphate. The same complex also shows high ability to inhibit β-haematin formation.

The mechanism of antimalarial action of $[Au(CQ)(PPh_3)]PF_6$ has been clearly defined [22]. Structural effects and increased drug lipophilicity enhance haem aggregation inhibition at lipid/water interfaces [24].

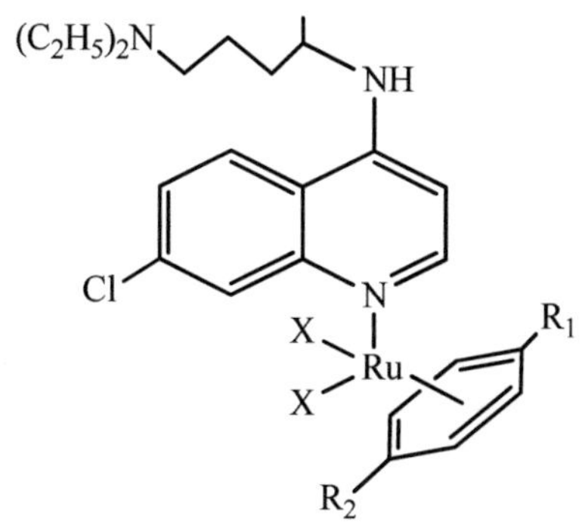

1. R_1 = $-CH_3$, R_2 = $-CH(CH_3)_2$, X = Cl^-

2. R_1=R_2 = H, X = Cl^-

Compound	CQ-Sensitive strains	CQ-Resistance strains	Reference
6	FcB1, 3D7, PFB, F32	W2, Dd2, K1	[25]
7	FcB1, 3D7, PFB, F32	W2, Dd2, K1	[25]

The description of CQ derivatives with Arene–metal complexes and half-sandwich complexes are shown above, where some of them showed high antiplamodial activity and some showed different modes of binding with CQ.

Ferroquine (FQ) shows higher biological and structural activity than any other antimalarial drugs in the market including chloroquine (CQ). The reaction of FQ and CQ against *P.*

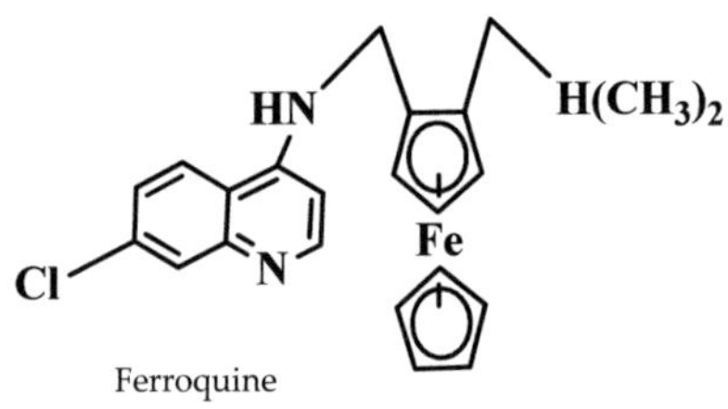

Ferroquine

falciparum strains is quite unique and different in which FQ reveal some high potency in chloroquine-resistant and chloroquine-sensitive *P. falciparum* strains[26-32].

Indeed it has been observed that a number of drugs that are active against CQ-resistant strains, including metal-based CQ derivatives, such as the iron-containing ferroquine [21,28,33] and the gold-CQ complex [Au(CQ)(PPh3)]PF6 [34], are considerably more lipophilic than CQ and this could be an important factor in the reduction of resistance.

Antiplasmodial activity of the synthetic products of chloroquine-bridged ferrocenophane analogues of ferroquine were reported by Salas *et. al.* (2013) [35]. All the disubstituted bridged ferrocenyl compounds were observed to be active against all the tested parasite strains.

The activities of some of the compounds under investigation were observed to be sensitive to the drug resistance level of the parasite strains. It was noted that:

- FQ was twenty times or more potent or operative against chloroquine-resistant parasite strains than CQ;
- FQ also displayed high level of potency *in vivo* in some experiments against *P. berghei, P. vinckei* and *P. yoeli;*
- Due to the different formulation and structure, there were no expected differences.

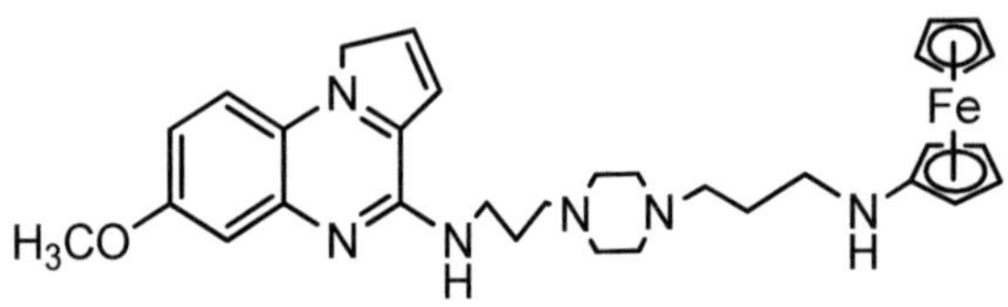

ferrocene–pyrrolo[1,2-α]quinoxaline compounds

This drug has shown lower resistance than chloroquine, therefore making their derivatives a good contender for chloroquine-resistant malaria. [36]. The most potent of this derivative contains a methoxy group just like the above.

Compound	CQ-Sensitive strains	CQ-Resistance strains	Reference
F	F32	FcB1, PFB	[36]

4. Multiple drug resistance mechanisms in cancer

The process and system whereby resistance to one drug is accompanied by resistance to drugs whose structures and mechanisms of action may be completely different is called multiple drug resistance (MDR). [37-42]

4.1. Platinum anticancer agents

One of the most effectively used drugs in cancer and for its treatment is the family called Platinium (II) complexes. The following compounds have been clinically approved for treatment universally.

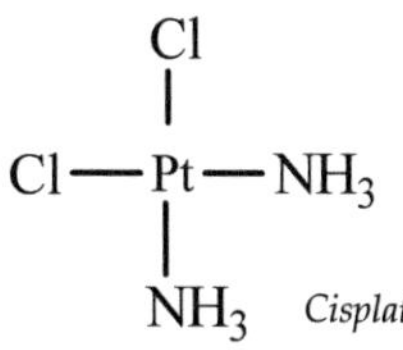

Cisplatin

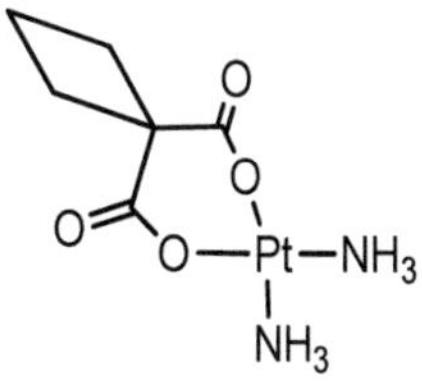

Carboplatin

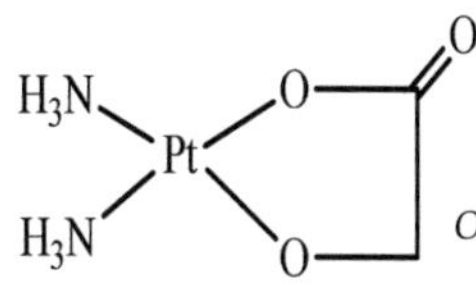

Oxaliplatin

Consideration of the toxic reduction of platinum complexes in living cells has been of special interest over the years. This happened so as to have a wider range of cure over other types of cancer that have come to light, hereby avoiding being stopped by some resistance. [43-45]

The usefulness of Platinum complexes in the clinical stage is limited by:

i. the spectrum of its anticancer activity (not active enough against several types of cancer),

ii. the development of resistance after continued treatment, and

iii. its high toxicity to some normal cells.

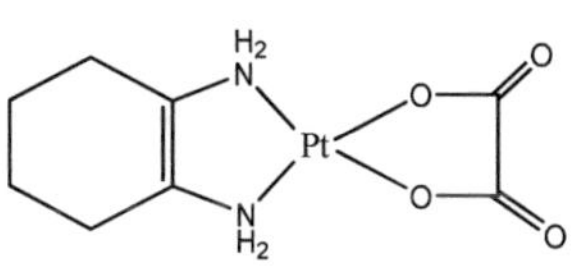

Oxaliplatin

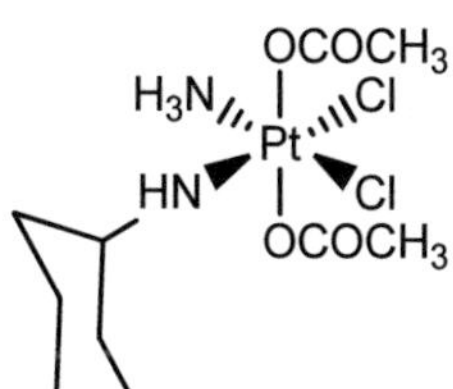

JM216

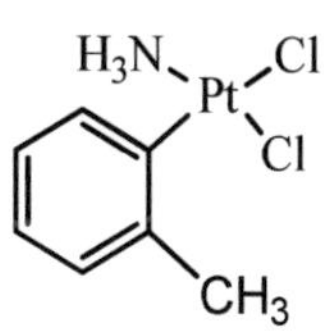

AMD473

Some of the current thinking on the chemical basis for the mechanism of action of cisplatin as an anticancer drug is summarized below:

In 2000, Pe´rez *et. al.* [46], were able to report the first crystal structure of a biologically active *trans*-platinum compound *trans*-[$PtCl_2$(dimethylamine)(isopropylamine) containing different

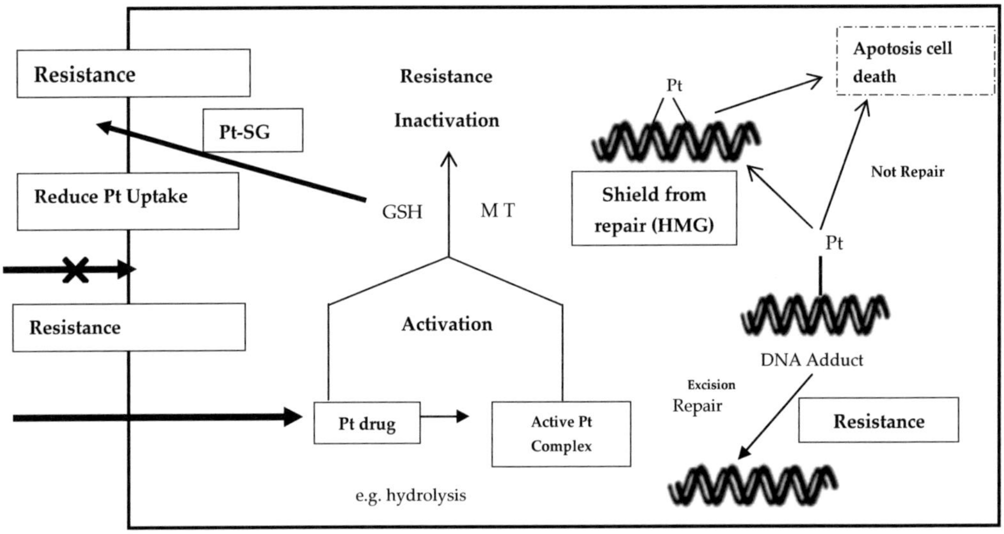

Figure 1. A summary of some of the processes that are thought to be involved in the cytotoxicity of platinum anticancer agents

aliphatic amines where *trans*-$PtCl_2$(dimethylamine)-(isopropylamine)] readily form DNA inter-stand crosslinks.

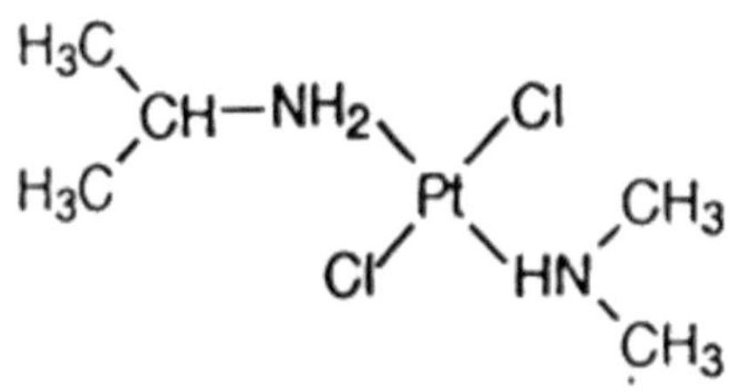

Trans-[$PtCl_2$(dimethylamine)(isopropylamine)]

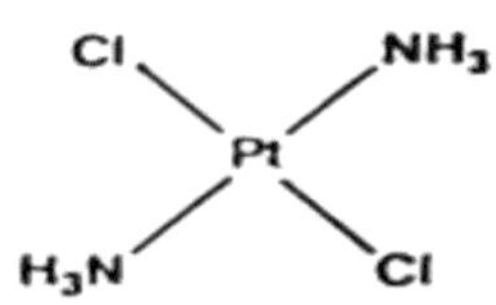

Transplatin

*tra*CC)(Cisopropy Transplatin lamincce)

But in the year 2003, Ramos-Lima *et al*, were able to replace two amine groups of transplatin with aliphatic amine and phosphane group, which resulted in circumvention of cisplatin resistance [47-48].

The synthesis pathway for the novel complexes is shown below;

http://dx.doi.org/10.5772/61033

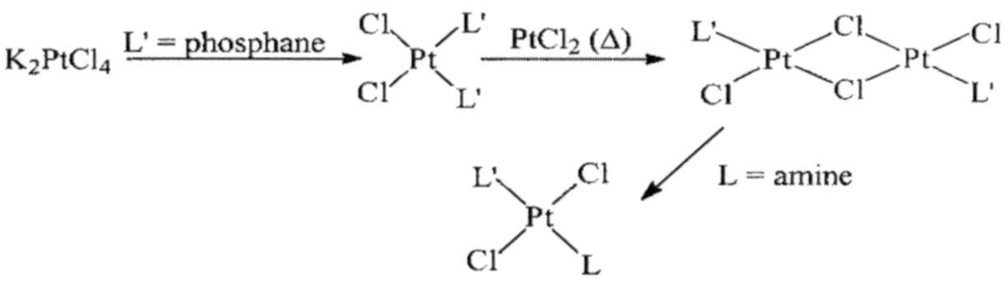

In 2014, Obaleye and co-workers synthesized and characterized a novel –M–X–M–X– type infinite chain 1D Cu(II) complex with eflornithine hydrochloride hydrate as ligand where their biological evaluation were examined and the results of the antibacterial screening show appreciable activity of the metal-drug complexes compared to the ligand when challenged with test organisms at varying concentrations. Copper complex was effective at virtually all concentrations used except against *E. coli* and *P. aeruginosa* at 0. 0001 gL^{-1} [49].

Highest susceptibility to Copper complex was recorded by S. aureus with clearance zone of 4. 2 mm at 1. 0 gL^{-1}. The results show that the metal-drug complex possesses a measure of antibacterial activity against all the organisms tested. The results also agree with the findings of other researchers [50-51] that antibacterial potency is usually concentration dependent.

The data also revealed that the activity of the Ligand EFL was bacteriostatic against all the organisms tested, while the activity of the copper (II) complex was bacteriostatic against *E. coli* and *P. aeruginosa* but bactericidal against S. aureus at 0. 0001 g/L concentration.

The Scheme of the reaction is shown below:

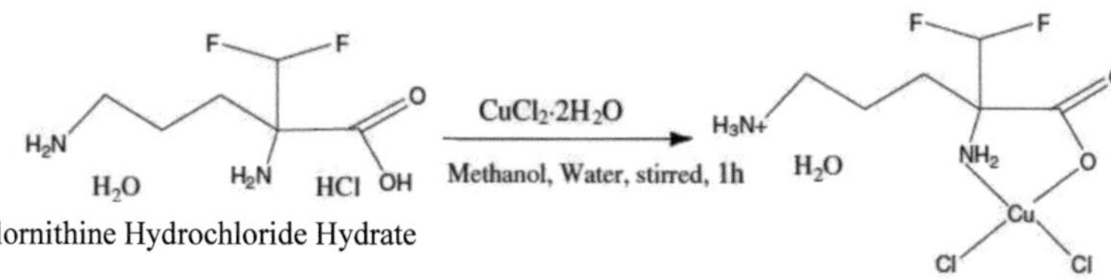

Eflornithine Hydrochloride Hydrate

Ligand EFL

5. Conclusion

For a couple of years now, some bacteria are becoming resistant to antibiotic drugs during this era of chemotherapy. This has been the main cause of morbidity and mortality worldwide. Many reasons had been attached to this drug resistance of the organism. Some of these proposed reasons are (i) the over-prescription of the drugs by physicians,(ii) self-medication, (iii) premature discontinuity of the medication by the patients as they start to regain strength and (iv) difficulty in affording the full course of the therapy. Other factors such as the transmission of the drug-resistant organism among patients through air or by direct contact with contaminated person or environment have been identified. It is also attested that a long period is usually needed to complete the treatment of individuals infected by the organisms. Modes of action of some of the potent antibiotic drugs are sometimes tagged as unknown. Hence, there is urgent need for continuous research in the development of drugs in order to have more effective drugs than the already available less potent drugs that will combat these dangerous microbes.

Although several metal-drug complexes have been synthesized to date, there are few of them at the final clinical stage due to their resistance capacity. Many researches are ongoing to circumvent this drug resistance, from this review, it is clear that some of the existing organic ligands or their derivatives are observed to be more potent when complexed with metals. These metal-drug complexes are *in vitro* and *in vivo* efficient.

In the aspect of antimalarial, antitumor, and anticancer drugs, more profitable researches are gradually emerging, yielding positive products with decent potency, stability, and reduced side effects. In this review resistance mechanisms of some synthesized metal-drug complexes were highlighted based on the investigations of various researchers.

Acknowledgements

The authors are grateful to Science and Technology Education Post–Basic Project (Step B) for their support and the University of Ilorin and for awarding of a Senate Rresearch grant.

Author details

Joshua A. Obaleye[1*], Nzikahyel Simon[2], Olufunso O. Abosede[1], Mercy O. Bamigboye[3], Abiodun A. Ajibola[1], Uche B. Eke[1] and Elizabeth A. Balogun[4]

*Address all correspondence to: jobaleye@unilorin.edu.ng

1 Department of Chemistry, University of Ilorin, Ilorin, Kwara State, Nigeria

2 Department of Chemistry, University of Uyo, Uyo, Akwa Ibom State, Nigeria

3 Department of Industrial Chemistry, University of Ilorin, Ilorin, Kwara State, Nigeria

4 Department of Biochemistry, University of Ilorin, Ilorin, Kwara State, Nigeria

References

[1] Saeed, A.; Najma, S.; Urooj, H.; and Ahmed Mesaik, M. (2009) Synthesis, characterization, antibacterial and anti-inflammatory activities of Enoxacin metal complexes. Bioinorganic chemistry and applications BioinorgChem Appl.,2009 : 6.

[2] Shi, R.; Itagaki, N.; and Sugawara, I. (2007). Overview of anti-tuberculosis(TB) drugs and their resistance mechanisms. Mini-Reviews in Medicinal Chemistry, 7:1177-1185.

[3] Heifets, L. B. (1994). Antimycobacterial drugs. Seminars in Respiratory Infections, 9(2):84.

[4] Bartmann, K. (1998). Isoniazid: In anti-tuberculosis drugs: Handbook of Experimental Pharmacology, Bartmann, K. Ed.; Springer-verlag, Berlin, pp. 113-134.

[5] Bardon, F.; Raynaud, C.; and Ramos, C. (1998). Microbiology, 144:2539-2543.

[6] Zhang, Y.; Heym, B.; Allen, B.; Young, D.; and Cole, S. T. (1992). The catalase- peroxidase gene and isoniazid resistance of Mycobacterium tuberculosis. Nature, 358(6387)591-593.

[7] Stoeckle, M. Y.; Guan, L.; Riegler, N.; Weitzman, I.; Kreiswirth, B.; Kornblum, J.; Laraque, F.; and Riley, L. W. (1993). Catalase-peroxidase gene sequences in isoniazid-sensitive and -resistant strains of Mycobacterium tuberculosis from New York City. J. Infect. Dis.;168(4):1063-5.

[8] Sensi, P. (1983). Antituberculosis drugs: Mechanisms of action and research trends. Rev. Infect. Dis. 30(Suppl. 3):24-28.

[9] Lippard, S. J. Metals in Medicine Department of Chemistry, Massachusetts Institute of Technology.

[10] Martell, A. E. (ed.),(1980) 'Inorganic Chemistry in Biology and Medicine', American Chemical Sot. Symposium, Series 8 140, Washington D. C.

[11] Klofutar, C.; Palik, S.; and Krasovec, I.; and Suhac, P. (1976) Kern. 9 Ind., 24, 361 (1975); Chem. Abstr., 84, 84739.

[12] Burchenal J. H. (1978), Biochemie, 60, 915.

[13] Thompson A. J. (1974) 'Platinum Coordination Complexes in Cancer Chemotherapy', Springer-Verlag, New York, p. 38

[14] WHO (2006). Guidelines for the treatment of malaria, Global Malaria Programme, 2nd edition. Geneva 1- 210

[15] Roper, C.; Pearce, R.; Nair, S.; Sharp, B.; Nosten, F.; and Andersson, T. (2004) Intercontinental spread of pyrimethamine–resistant malaria, Science, 305(5687): 1124

[16] Bray, R. S.; and Garnham, P. C. (1982) The life-cycle of primate malaria parasites. Br. Med. Bull. 38, 117–122.

[17] Petersen, I.; Eastman, R.; and Lanzer, M. (2011) 1551–1562 Drug-resistant malaria: Molecular mechanisms and implications for public health.

[18] Sanchez-Delgado, R. A.; and Anzellotti, A. (2004) Metal complexes as chemotherapeutic agents against tropical diseases: trypanosomiais, malaria and leishmaniasis. Mini Rev. Med. Chem. 4, 23–30

[19] Sharma, V. (2005) Therapeutic drugs for targeting chloroquine resistance in malaria. Mini Rev. Med. Chem. 5, 337–351

[20] Navarro, M. (2009) Gold complexes as potential anti-parasitic agents. Coord. Chem.

[21] Rev. 253, 1619–1626

[22] Sánchez-Delgado, R. A.; Navarro, M.; Perez, H.; Urbina, J. A. (1996) J. Med. Chem. 39, 1095.

[23] Navarro, M.; Perez, H.; Sánchez-Delgado, R. A. (1997). J. Med. Chem. 40, 1937.

[24] Navarro, M.; Vasquez, F.; Sánchez-Delgado, R. A.; Perez, H.; Sinou, V.; Schrevel, J. (2004). J. Med. Chem. 47, 5204.

[25] Navarro M.; Castro W.; Martínez A., Sánchez Delgado R. A. (2011); J. Inorg. Biochem. 105, 276–282

[26] Rajapakse, C. S. K.; Martínez, A.; Naoulou, B.; Jarzecki, A. A.; Suarez, L.; Deregnaucourt, C.; Sinou, V.; Schrevel, J.; Musi, E.; Ambrosini, G.; Schwartz, G. K.; Sánchez-Delgado, R. A. (2009) Inorg. Chem., 48, 1122.

[27] Biot, C.; Glorian, G.; Maciejewski, L. A.; Brocard, J. S.; Domarle, O.; Blampain, G.; Millet, P.; Georges, A. J.; Abessolo, H.; Dive, D.; Lebibi, J. (1997) J. Med. Chem., 40, 3715.

[28] Domarle, O.; Blampain, G.; Agnaniet, H.; Nzadiyabi, T.; Lebibi, J.; Brocard, J.; Maciejewski, L.; Biot, C.; Georges, A. J.; Millet, P. (1998) Antimicrob. Agents Chemother. 42, 540.

[29] Biot, C.; Daher, W.; Ndiaye, C. M.; Melnyk, P.; Pradines, B.; Chavain, N.; Pellet, A.; Fraisse, L.; Pelinski, L.; Jarry, C.; Brocard, J.; Khalife, J.; Forfar-Bares, I. (2006); Dive, D. J. Med. Chem., 49, 4707.

[30] Beagley, P.; Blackie, M. A. L.; Chibale, K.; Clarkson, C.; Moss, J. R.; Smith, P. J. (2002), J. Chem. Soc., Dalton Trans., 23, 4426.

[31] Pradines, B.; Fusai, T.; Daries, W.; Laloge, V.; Rogier, C.; Millet, P.; Panconi, E.; Kombila, M.; Parzy, D. (2001), J. Antimicrob. Chemother., 48, 179.

[32] Blackie, M. A. L.; Beagley, P.; Croft, S. L.; Kendrick, H.; Moss, J. R.; Chibale, K. (2007) Bioorg. Med. Chem., 15, 6510.

[33] Beagley, P.; Blackie, M. A. L.; Chibale, K.; Clarkson, C.; Meijboom, R.; Moss, J. R.; Smith, P. J.; Su, H. (2003) Dalton Trans., 15, 3046.

[34] Biot, C. (2004) Curr Med Chem Anti-Infect Agents; 3:135–147.

[35] Biot, C.; Tarameli, D.; Forfar-Bares, I.; Maciejewski, L. A.; Boyce, M.; Nowogrocki, G.; Brocard, J. S.; Basilico, N.; Olliaro, P., Egan T. J. (2005) Mol. Pharm. 2:185–193. [PubMed: 15934779]

[36] Salas, P. F.; Herrmann, C.; Cawthray, J. F.; Nimphius, C.; Kenkel, A.; Chen, J.; Carmen de Kock; Smith, P. J.; Patrick, B. O.; Adam, M. J.; and Orvig, C. (2013). Structural Characteristics of Chloroquine-Bridged Ferrocenophane Analogues of Ferroquine May Obviate Malaria Drug-Resistance Mechanisms. J. Med. Chem. 56(4), 1596-1613.

[37] Guillon, J.; Moreau, S.; Mouray, E.; Sinou, V.; Forfar, I.; Fabre, S. B.; Desplat, V.; Millet, P.; Parzy, D.; Jarry, C.; Grellier, P. (2008). Bioorg. Med. Chem. 16, 9133.

[38] Bolhuis, H.; Van Veen, H. W.; Poolman, B.; Driessen, A. J.; and Konings, W. N. (1997). Mechanisms of multidrug transporters. FEMS Microbiology Reviews, 21, 55–84.

[39] Kawase, M.; and Motohashi, N. (2003). New multidrug resistance reversal agents. Current Drug Targets, 4, 31–43.

[40] Szakacs, G.; Paterson, J. K.; Ludwig, J. A.; Booth-Genthe, C.; and Gottesman, M. M. (2006). Targeting multidrug resistance in cancer. Nature Reviews Drug Discovery, 5, 219–234.

[41] Ozben, T. (2006). Mechanisms and strategies to overcome multiple drug resistance in cancer. FEBS Letters, 580, 2903–2909.

[42] Dubikovskaya, E. A.; Thorne, S. H.; Pillow, T. H.; Contag, C. H.; and Wender, P. A. (2008). Overcoming multidrug resistance of small-molecule therapeutics through conjugation with releasable octaarginine transporters. Proceedings of the National Academy of Sciences of the United States of America, 105, 12128–12133.

[43] Baguley, B. C. (2010). Multidrug resistance in cancer. Methods in Molecular Biology, 596, 1–14.

[44] Abrams, M. J.; and Murrer, B. A. (1993) Science 261, 725-730.

[45] Kidani, Y.; Kizu, R.; Miyazaki, M.; Noji, M.; Matsuzawa A.; Takeda Y.; Akiyama N.; and Eriguchi, M. (1993) Platinum and Other Metal Coordination Compounds in Cancer Chemotherapy 2. H. M. Pinedo and J. H. Schornagel, eds., Plenum Press, New York, p43-51.

[46] Smith, C. A.; Sutherland-Smith, A. J.; Keppler, B. K.; Kratz, F.; and Baker E. N. (1996). J. Biol. Inorg. Chem. 1,424-431.

[47] Pe′rez, J. M.; Montero, E. I.; Gonzalez, A. M.; Solans, X.; Font-Bardia M. A.; Fuertes M. A., Alonso, C.; Navarro-Ranninger C. (2000), J. Med. Chem., 43, 2411-2418.

[48] Montero, E. I.; Dı′az, S.; Gonza′lez-Vadillo, A. M; Pe′rez J. M., Alonso C., Navarro-Ranninger C. (1999), J. Med. Chem. 42, 4264-4268.

[49] Francisco, J.; Ramos-Lima, A.; Quiroga, G.; Pe´rez, J. M.; Font-Bardı´a M, Solans X.; and Navarro-Ranninger C. (2003) Eur. J. Inorg. Chem., 1591-1598.

[50] Obaleye, J. A.; Tella, A. C.; Osunniran, W. A; Simon, N.; Omojasola, P. F; (2014). Synthesis, Characterization, Crystal Structure and Antimicrobial Evaluation of a Novel –M–X–M–X– Type Infinite Chain 1D Cu(II) Complex with Eflornithine Hydrochloride Hydrate as Ligand. 24: 827-835.

[51] Ekwenye, U. N.; Elegalam, N. N. (2005), J. Mol. Med. Adv. Sci. 1(4), 410.

[52] Omojasola P. F.; and Awe S. (2004), Biosci. Res. Comm. 16, 25.

Section 2

The Compounds

Chapter 3

Quinolone Compounds with Activity Against Multidrug-Resistant Gram-Positive Microorganisms

Pintilie Lucia

Additional information is available at the end of the chapter

http://dx.doi.org/10.5772/60948

Abstract

The emergence of resistance to antimicrobial agents is a global public health problem. Some microorganisms may develop resistance to a single antimicrobial agent (or related class of agent), while others develop resistance to several antimicrobial agents or classes. These organisms are often referred to as multidrug-resistant or MDR strains. Identification of new molecules that show activity against multidrug-resistant microorganisms and its development on a new antimicrobial drug, would be an important step in the fight against antimicrobial resistance. This paper presents experimental data regarding the synthesis of several quinolones. The novel compounds having quinolone structure were synthesized by Gould-Jacobs method. Their structure has been determined and confirmed by the following physicochemical methods: elemental analysis, IR spectral analysis, H-NMR, C-NMR, UV, thin layer chromatography. The new compounds have been evaluated for „in vitro" activity by determining minimum inhibitory concentration against a variety of bacteria Some of new quinolones, which showed a good activity, have been tested against 30 strains of methicillin resistant Staphylococcus aureus isolated in the Microbiology Laboratory of INBI Prof. "Dr. Matei Bals" during 2012 The minimum inhibitory concentration (MIC) of the isolates have been determined by agar plate Mueller Hinton (bioMerieux) dilution method using the reference strain Staphylococcus aureus ATCC 29213. The 30 strains of isolated have been also tested for susceptibility to ciprofloxacin, levofloxacin and imipenem by Etest method. Base on the "in vitro" studies, the quinolone FPQ-30 appears to be an promising compound, all strains isolates were inhibited at a concentration of 8 μg/ml.

Keywords: Quinolones, fluoroquinolones, antimicrobial agents, Methicillin-resistant Sthaphilococcus aureus

1. Introduction

The emergence of resistance to antimicrobial agents is a global public health problem. Some microorganisms may develop resistance to a single antimicrobial agent (or a related class of agents), while others develop resistance to several antimicrobial agents or classes. These organisms are often referred to as multidrug-resistant or MDR strains. Identification of new molecules that show activity against multidrug-resistant microorganisms and its development into a new antimicrobial drug would be an important step in the fight against antimicrobial resistance.

The discovery of fluoroquinolones after 1980 represented a decisive step forward for chemical anti-infectious therapy. A large number of fluoroquinolones are used today in medical practices and some of them are deemed by leading pharmacologists to be of vital importance to anti-infectious therapy.

2. Tendencies and strategies in the field of quinolones

The basic structure of quinolones (Figure 1) [9], is a bicyclic structure that contains a ring type A 4-pyridinone combined with an aromatic or heteroaromatic ring B. According to the nature of atoms symbolized by X, Y, Z, they can be defined as four subfamilies: naphthyridine 1-8, cinnoline, pyrido-2,3-pyrimidines, and quinolone.

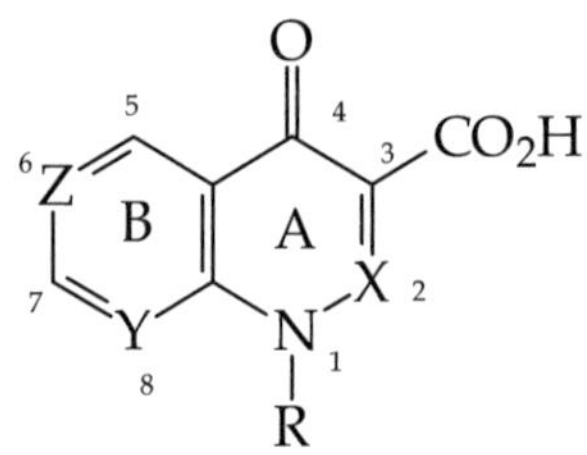

naphthyridines : X=Z=H; Y=N
cinnolin: X=N; Y=Z=H
pyrido-2,3-pyrimidine: X=H; Y=Z=N
quinolones : X=Y=Z= H

Figure 1. Basic structure of quinolones.

The structural modifications of the core of the quinolone influence the antimicrobial activity

2.1. Position 1

Research has been oriented in several directions:

- Introducing an unsubstituted or substituted alkyl: R_1 = methyl [32], ethyl [32, 28], *iso*propyl [28, 48, 1], *tert*-butyl [48, 14], fluoroethyl [28], hydroxyethyl [38], chloroethyl [38];
- Introduction of a vinyl, allyl [38, 32];
- Introduction of alkylamino groups [65];
- Introduction of a cyclpopropyl [38, 56, 57, 49] or cyclobutyl [49, 1];
- Introducing mono or disubstituted phenyl [38, 7, 46, 49];
- Introduction of a five-membered aromatic heterocycles: pyrrolyl, [34].

Usually, the most active compounds contain the ethyl substituent in position 1. Using a STERIMOL program, Fujita (1984), based on a set of five parameters that characterize the shape and size of a substituent and following a quantitative analysis of the relationship between chemical structure and biological activity on a set of N-1 allyl and alkyl derivatives have deduced the optimum length of the substituent in position 1 is 0.42 nm [9, 58], which corresponds to the ethyl substituent. In general, the most active components contain in position 1 an ethyl substituent. These studies have already been confirmed by the results achieved with quinolones that are used in therapeutic practice: nalidixic acid, oxolinic acid, norfloxacin, pefloxacin, quinolones that have an ethyl substituent in N-1 position.

In Table 1 is presented the antimicrobial activity for the 1-substituted quinolones against gram positive and gram negative microorganisms. By comparison, data are entered for norfloxacin (R_1 = ethyl) and ciprofloxacin (R_1 = c-C_3H_5).

Replacing ethyl substituent with:

- Sterically comparable substituents (2-fluoroethyl and vinyl) lead to compounds with comparable activity on gram negative bacteria, while replacing with substituent steric hindrance effect more or less pronounced (methyl, 2 hydroxy-ethyl, n-propyl, allyl, benzyl, cyclopropyl-methyl) leads to decreased activity of "in vitro".
- *Tert*-butyl substituent leads to compounds that possess good antimicrobial activity against *Staphylococcus aureus*, while against gram negative microorganisms, the activity is comparable to the reference compound (norfloxacin). Increasing the number of carbon atoms (number of carbon atoms > 4) results in decreased antimicrobial activity. The replacement of a hydrogen by fluorine atom leads to the increase of antibacterial activity two to three times compared to the compound where R_1 = *tert*-butyl, while introducing more fluorine atoms leads to a decrease in the antimicrobial activity.

In series N-1 cyclopropyl (ciprofloxacin), the substituent from N-1 position has a larger volume than the ethyl. This is contrary to the concept of the steric volume. High antimicrobial activity of the ciprofloxacin may be caused by this hyperconjugation or self-association properties induced by the cyclopropyl. For compounds that present in this position, a cycloalkyl with a number of carbon atoms of more than 3 (cyclobutyl, cyclopentyl) the antimicrobial activity is much reduced compared to ciprofloxacin.

The following are relevant for the chemical structure–biological activity relationships:

- The nature of the substituent introduced in the alkyl moiety at N-1 position of quinolone: the fluorine atom has benefic influence on the antimicrobial activity;
- The position where the substituents are introduced in the alkyl moiety: substituents in position 1 of the alkyl moiety have positive influence on antimicrobial activity;
- The number of substituents placed on the alkyl moiety: increasing the number of substituents leads to decreased antimicrobial activity;
- Presence of cis-trans stereoisomers: cis derivatives are more active against gram positive bacteria than the trans derivatives, while the activity is comparable against gram negative bacteria.

Relevant for the chemical structure–biological activity relationships are to:

- Nature of the substituent introduced in the alkyl moiety at N-1 position of quinolone: the fluorine atom has benefic influence on the antimicrobial activity;
- The position where the substituents are introduced in the alkyl moiety: substituents in position 1 of the alkyl moiety have positive influence on antimicrobial activity;
- The number of substituents placed on the alkyl moiety: increasing the number of substituents leads to decreased antimicrobial activity;
- Presence of cis-trans stereoisomers: cis derivatives are more active against gram positive bacteria than the trans derivatives, while the activity is comparable against gram negative bacteria.

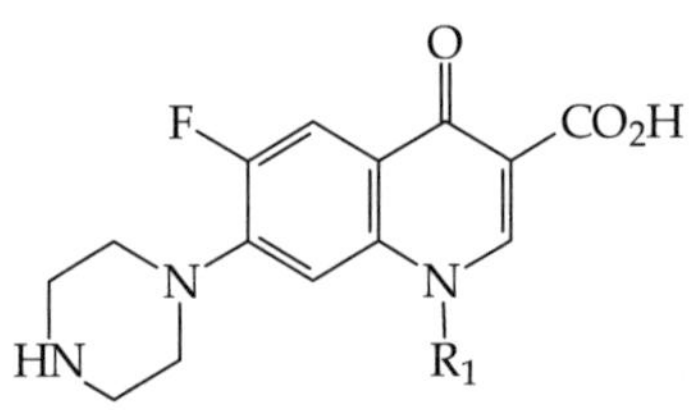

Figure 2. Quinolones with an aliphatic substituent in N-1 position.

R_1	Minimum inhibitory concentration (μg/ml)			Reference
	S. aureus	*E. coli*	*P. aeruginosa*	
$-CH_3$	6.25	0.39	1.56	(Koga et al. 1980)
$-C_2H_5$ (Norfloxacin)	0.39	0.05	0.39	(Koga et al. 1980)
$-CH=CH_2$	3.13	0.10	0.39	(Koga et al. 1980)
$n-C_3H_7$	1.56	0.20	3.13	(Koga et al. 1980)

http://dx.doi.org/10.5772/60948

R_1	Minimum inhibitory concentration (μg/ml)			Reference
	S. aureus	*E. coli*	*P. aeruginosa*	
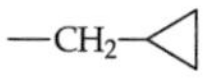	1.00	0.50	4.00	(Bouzard et al. 1989)
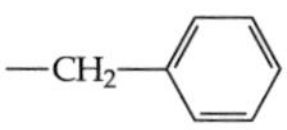	1.56	0.78	1.56	(Koga et al. 1980) (Bouzard et al. 1989)
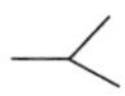	1.00	0.50	1.00	(Bouzard et al. 1989)
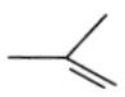	0.50	0.13	0.50	(Bouzard et al. 1989)
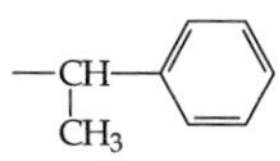	4.00	2.00	32.00	(Bouzard et al. 1989)
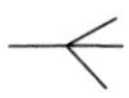	0.25	0.06	0.50	(Remuzon et al. 1991)
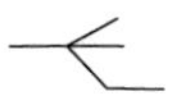	0.25	0.50	4.00	(Bouzard et al. 1989)
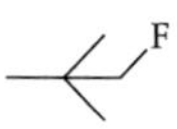	0.13	0.016	0.25	(Remuzon et al. 1991)
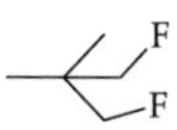	1.00	0.13	1.00	(Remuzon et al. 1991)
$-CH_2CH_2F$	1.56	0.10	0,.78	(Koga et al. 1980)
$-CH_2CH_2OH$	1.56	0.39	3.13	(Koga et al. 1980)
$-NH-CH_3$	1.95	1.00	1.00	(Koga et al. 1980) (Wentland et al. 1984)
$-CH_2-CH=CH_2$	3.13	0.20	1.56	(Koga et al. 1980)
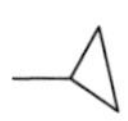 (Ciprofloxacin)	0.13	0.03	0.013	(Chu&Fernandes 1991)
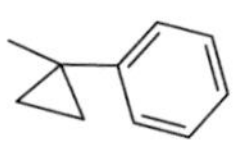	0.13	0.13	4.00	(Bouzard et al. 1989)
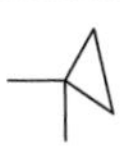	0.25	0.06	0.50	(Bouzard et al. 1989)

R$_1$	Minimum inhibitory concentration (μg/ml)			Reference
	S. aureus	*E. coli*	*P. aeruginosa*	
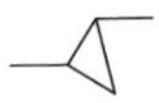 (trans)	1.00	0.06	2.00	(Bouzard et al. 1989)
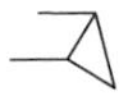 (cis)	0.13	0.13	1.00	(Bouzard et al. 1989)
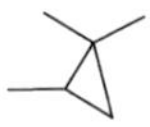	1.00	1.00	32.00	(Bouzard et al. 1989)
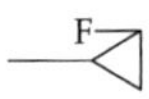 (cis)	0.10	≤0.05	≤0.05	(Youichi et al. 1994) (Shongo et al. 1993)
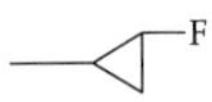 (trans)	0.78	≤0.05	0.10	(Youichi et al. 1994) (Shongo et al. 1993)
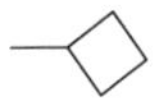	0.50	0.13	1.00	(Bouzard et al. 1989)
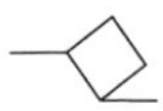	4.00	2.00	32.00	(Bouzard et al. 1989)
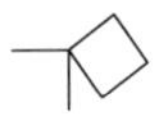	0.50	0.25	8.00	(Bouzard et al. 1989)
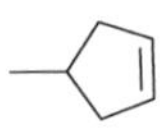	2.00	1.00	8.00	(Bouzard et al. 1989)
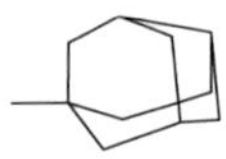	8.00	2.00	63.00	(Bouzard et al. 1989)

Table 1. MIC values (μg/ml) for quinolones with an aliphatic substituent in N-1 position

It is obvious that the volume of the substituent at position N-1 is not the only factor influencing the antibacterial activity of the quinolones. There are other factors that have a considerable influence on biological activity such as, for example, the effects of conjugation, conformational effects. This has been demonstrated by the synthesis of compounds containing aryl substituents in N-1 position [32, 7, 8, 46].

In Table 2 are presented data on the antimicrobial activity of 7-piperazinyl and 7- (4-methyl-piperazinyl)-quinolone derivatives having substituted or unsubstituted aryl substituents in N-1 position.

http://dx.doi.org/10.5772/60948

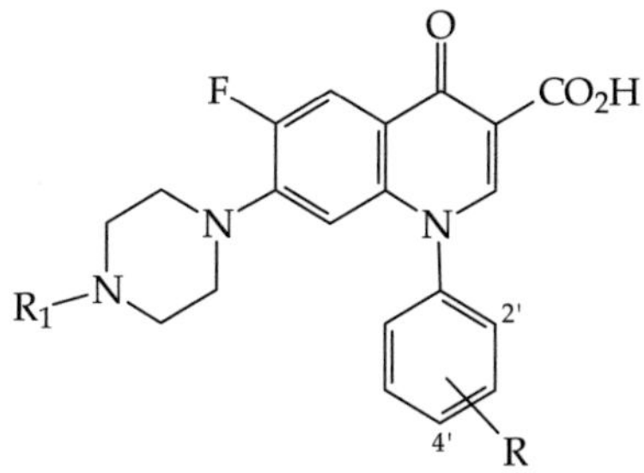

Figure 3. Aryl-quinolones.

Compound	R	R_1	Minimum inhibitory concentration (μg/ ml)			Reference
			S. areus	*E. coli*	*P. aeruginosa*	
Norfloxacin			0.39	0.05	0.39	2
1	H	H	0.20	0.78	0.78	(Chu et al. 1985)
Sarafloxacin	4-F	H	0.20	0.05	0.39	(Chu et al. 1985)
2	H	CH_3	0.78	0.78	6.20	(Chu et al. 1985)
3	2-F	CH_3	1.56	0.78	6.20	(Chu et al. 1985)
4	3-F	CH_3	12.50	6.20	50.00	(Chu et al. 1985)
Difloxacin	4-F	CH_3	0.20	0.20	1.56	(Chu et al. 1985)
5	4-Br	CH_3	3.10	6.20	50.00	(Chu et al. 1985)
6	4-Cl	CH_3	1.56	1.56	12.50	(Chu et al. 1985)
7	4-OH	CH_3	0.05	0.10	0.39	(Chu et al. 1985)
8	4-OCH_3	CH_3	1.,50	50.00	200.00	(Chu et al. 1985)
9	4-CH_3	CH_3	1.56	1.56	12.50	(Chu et al. 1985)
10	3,4-OCH_2O-	CH_3	0.75	0.78	6.20	(Chu et al. 1985)
11	2-F,4v-F	CH_3	0.10	0.20	1.56	(Chu et al. 1985)
12	2'-CH_3	CH_3	3.10	1.56	25.00	(Chu et al. 1985)
13	2-CH_3,4CH_3	CH_3	100.00	100.00	100.00	(Chu et al. 1985)
14	4-NO_2	CH_3	64.00	8.00	128.00	(Radl & Zikan 1989)
15	4-NH_2	CH_3	2.00	1.00	32.00	(Radl & Zikan 1989)

Table 2. The "in vitro"" antibacterial activity of 1-aryl-quinolones

For *7-piperazinyl quinolones,* the introduction of an unsubstituted aryl affords a compound (compound 1 – Table 2) with good antimicrobial activity "in vitro" against *S. aureus* being more active than the reference compound, norfloxacin.

The presence of a substituent on the aryl nucleus leads to improved antimicrobial activity, e.g. a fluorine atom (sarafloxacina) in the 4-position of the phenyl ring.

In the series 7-(4-methyl-piperazinyl)-1-aryl-quinolones the best results are obtained when in position 4 is located a fluorine atom (for example, difloxacin) or -OH (compound 7). Good results are also obtained in the case of two substituents present (positions 2 and 4) on the aryl nucleus (R = F) (compound 11).

2.2. Position 2

Some changes were explored for this position [9]. Replacing the carbon atom of oxolinic acid with a nitrogen atom (which led to cinoxacin) has resulted in improved pharmacokinetic properties, but has led to decreased antimicrobial activity "in vitro". Significant reductions in bacterial activity were also observed in the case of 2-aza-4-quinolones derivatives from norfloxacin and pefloxacin. The introduction of substituents on the carbon atom in position 2, for example, hydroxy, methyl, methylthio, etc., leads to the inactivation of the quinolone compounds.

2.3. Position 3

In the quinolone molecule, combination between carboxyl group from 3 position and ketone group in 4 position, is considered necessary for binding to DNA gyrasa, while the presence of carboxyl group in 3 position is essential for antimicrobial activity. Modification of carboxyl groups, generally leads to obtaining biologically inactive compounds (Figure 4) [62]. The exceptions are groups that can be converted "in vitro" to the carboxyl function.

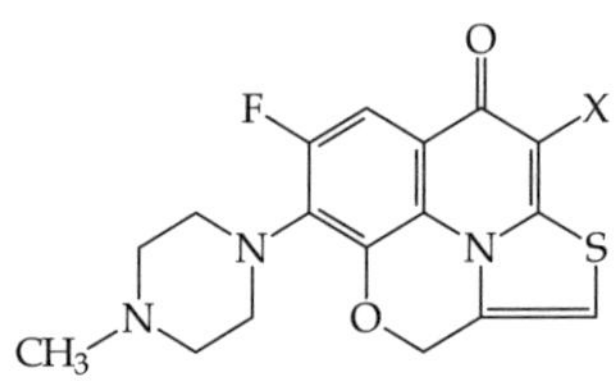

Figure 4. X = H, 4b: X = SO_3H

The researches regarding changes of the substituent in the 3 position of quinolone, followed to obtain:

- Compounds presenting free carboxyl group;
- Bioreversible compounds (prodrugs) ester (Figures 5, 6), [59, 51], which easily hydrolyzed in the body releasing the carboxyl group;

http://dx.doi.org/10.5772/60948

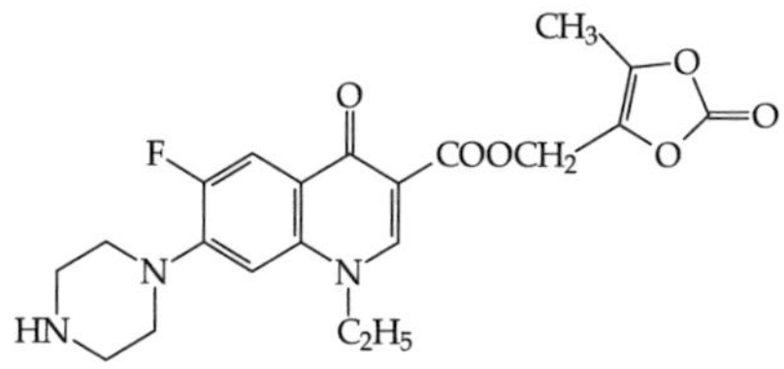

Figure 5. Methyl-2-oxo-1,3-dioxol-4-yl) ethyl ester

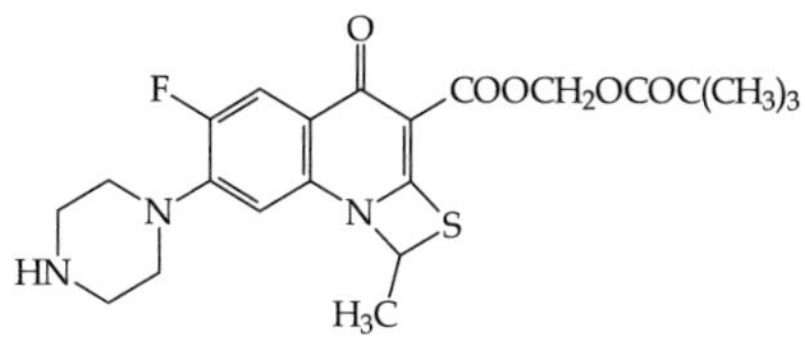

Figure 6. Pivaloiloxymethyl ester

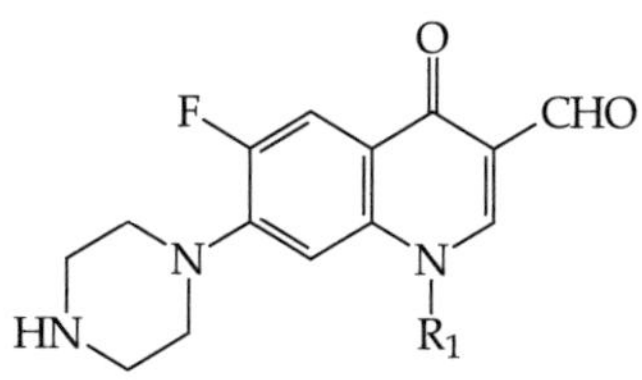

Figure 7. R_1 = ethyl, cyclopropyl, R = H, methyl

- Bioreversible derivatives (prodrugs) - 3-formyl-quinolone (Figure 7) [31];
- Quinoline-3-carboxamide: (Wetland et al. 1993), (Sajay et al. 2000).

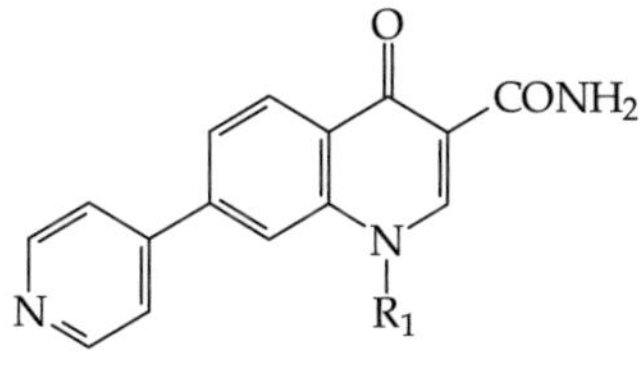

Figure 8. R_1 = alkyl, mono or disubstituted phenyl

Both types of structures (Figures 8 and 9) have been hydrolyzed in the body; carboxyl group has been generated; and through this the biological activity was explained, with the observation that the time to reach that MICs is greater.

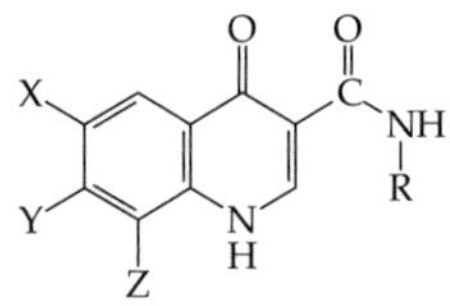

Figure 9. X = H,Cl,F,NO_2, Y = H,Cl,NO_2 Z = H,CH_3,F, R = cyclopropyl, n-octyl, (N, N-diethylamino-1-methyl) butyl

2.4. Position 4

The quinolone structure requires the presence of the ketone group in position 4. Replacing this ketone group, the 4-thiooxo or 4-sulfonyl groups led to obtaining inactive compounds [9].

2.5. Position 5

In position 5 of the quinolones various groups were introduced, such as nitro (Domagala et al. 1988) unsubstituted or substituted amino [27, 16, 36] [17], alkyl [23, 25], halogen [35, 36], mercapto [35, 36], hydroxy [36, 17], alkoxy or tioalcooxi [35, 36]

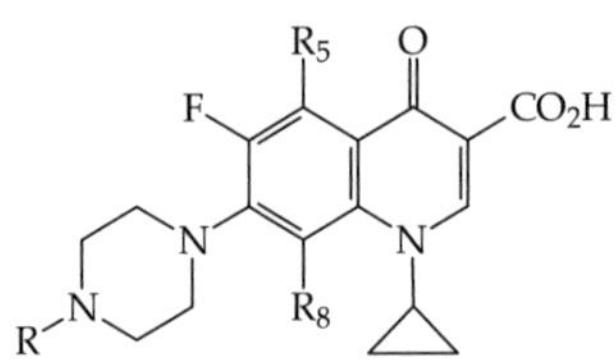

Figure 10. Substituted quinolones.

R	R_5	R_8	Minimum inhibitory concentration (μg/ml)			Reference
			S. aureus	*E. coli*	*P. aeruginosa*	
H	H	H	0.2	0.013	0.4	(Domagala et al.1991)(*)
H	NH_2	H	0.025	0.013	0.8	(Domagala et al.1991)(*)
H	NH_2	F	0.013 0.013 0.050	0.013 0.013 0.0063	0.025 0.025 0.1	(Domagala et al.1991)(*) (Domagala et al.1988)(*) (Myamoto et al. 1990) 74(**)
H	CH_3NH	F	0.2	0.1	1.6	(Domagala et al.1988)(*)
H	AcNH	F	>25	>25	>25	(Domagala et al.1988)(*)
H	NH_2	Cl	0.025	0.025	0.8	(Domagala et al.1991)(*)
H	HO	H	0.2	0.025	0.4	(Domagala et al.1991)(*)

http://dx.doi.org/10.5772/60948

R	R_5	R_8	Minimum inhibitory concentration (μg/ml)			Reference
			S. aureus	*E. coli*	*P. aeruginosa*	
H	HO	F	0.2 0.2	0.05 0.025	0.8 0.39	(Myamoto et al. 1990) (**)
H	CH_3	H	0.025	0.013	0.2	(Hagen et al. 1991) (*)
H	CH_3	F	0.025	0.025	0.2	(Hagen et al. 1991) (*)
H	CH_3	Cl	0.025	0.025	0.2	(Hagen et al. 1991) (*)
H	C_2H_5	H	6.30	0.4	12.5	(Hagen et al. 1991) (*)
H	F	F	0.2	0.0125	0.39	(Myamoto et al. 1990) (**)
H	Cl	F	0.1	0.0125	0.39	(Myamoto et al. 1990) (**)
CH_3	H	F	0.2	0.025	0.39	(Myamoto et al. 1990) (**)
CH_3	F	F	0.39	0.05	0.78	(Myamoto et al. 1990) (**)
CH_3	Cl	F	0.2	0.025	0.78	(Myamoto et al. 1990) (**)
CH_3	Br	F	0.39	0.05	0.78	(Myamoto et al. 1990) (**)
CH_3	HO	F	0.2	0.05	0.78	(Myamoto et al. 1990) (**)
CH_3	CH_3O	F	25	0.2	12.5	(Myamoto et al. 1990) (**)
CH_3	$PhCH_2O$	F	6.25	1.56	6.25	(Myamoto et al. 1990) (**)
CH_3	HS	F	3.13	0.39	12.5	(Myamoto et al. 1990) (**)
CH_3	CH_3S	F	3.13	0.2	12.5	(Myamoto et al. 1990) (**)
CH_3	4-CH_3OPhCH_2S	F	100	12.5	>100	(Myamoto et al. 1990) (**)
CH_3	NH_2	F	0.1 0.013	0,0125 0.025	0.2 0.1	(Domagala et al.1988)(*) (Myamoto et al. 1990) (**)
CH_3	CH_3NH	F	0.78	0.1	1.56	(Myamoto et al. 1990) (**)
CH_3	$(CH_3)_2N$	F	25 >25	3,.3 >25	50 >25	(Domagala et al.1988) (Myamoto et al. 1990) (**)
CH_3	$PhCH_2NH$	F	0.78	0.78	3.13	(Myamoto et al. 1990) (**)
CH_3	$HOCH_2CH_2NH$	F	0.39	0.5	0.78	(Myamoto et al. 1990) (**)
CH_3	$(CH_3)_2NCH_2CH_2NH$	F	6.25	0.05	0.78	(Myamoto et al. 1990) (**)
CH_3	pyrrolyl	F	3.13	0.39	12.5	(Myamoto et al. 1990) (**)

Ciprofloxacina ; * *S. aureus* UC 76 ; * *E. coli* Vogel; * *P. aeruginosa*.UI-18; ***S. aureus* 209P JC-1 ; ***E. coli* NIIHJ JC-2; ***P. aeriginosa* 12

Table 3. The "in vitro" antibacterial activity of 5-substituted quinolones

In the series of *1-cyclopropyl-7-piperazinyl quinolones*, the influence of the substituent in position 5 on the antimicrobial activity is manifested as follows:

- The introduction of unsubstituted amino group when $R_8 = H$ leads to increased antibacterial activity against gram positive only, while when $R_8 = F$ or Cl leads to the increase of antibacterial activity on gram positive and gram negative microorganisms.
- The introduction of substituted amino group leads to the lowering of antimicrobial activity on the entire microbial spectrum.
- The introduction of the hydroxy group (R_8 = H, F), does not produce any change in the antibacterial activity.
- The introduction of the methyl group (R_8 = H, F, Cl) causes increased activity on the entire microbial spectrum.
- The introduction of an alkyl radical having a carbon number greater than 2 leads to decreased antimicrobial activity.
- The introduction of a halogen atom:
- For $R_5 = F$ ($R_8 = F$) – the antimicrobial activity remains unchanged on the entire microbacterial spectrum.
- For $R_5 = F$ ($R_8 = F$) – antibacterial activity is improved against gram positive bacteria).

In the series of *1-cyclopropyl-7-(4-methyl-piperazinyl)-quinolones*, the influence of the substituent in position 5 on the antimicrobial activity is manifested as follows:

- The introduction of an unsubstituted amino group ($R_8 = F$) leads to increased antibacterial activity against gram positive and gram negative microorganisms; the alkylation of the amino group leads to the lowering of antimicrobial activity on the entire microbial spectrum, the decrease being dependent on the size of the alkyl group (especially dialkylating lead to a loss of antibacterial activity).
- The introduction of a halogen atom (fluorine or bromine) ($R_8 = F$) leads to the slight decrease of activity compared to the unsubstituted compound; the introduction of a chlorine atom decreases antibacterial activity only against *Pseudomonas aeruginosa.*
- The introduction of a hydroxy group does not modify the biological activity. The introduction of a methoxy or benzyloxy group leads to decreasing of the antimicrobial activity against all tested microorganisms.
- The introduction of a mercapto group leads to a considerable decrease of the antimicrobial activity on the entire microbial spectrum. The same decrease is found in the case of methylthio group.
- The presence of a bulky substituent leads to the loss of biological activity against all microorganisms tested.

http://dx.doi.org/10.5772/60948

2.5.1. *In conclusion*

In the case of 1-cyclopropyl-7-piperazinyl-quinolones, antibacterial activity increases according to the nature of the substituent in position 5, in the following order:

For $R_8 = H : RO < HO < NH_2 < CH_3$;

For $R_8 = F : HO \leq F \leq Cl < CH_3 < F$

In the case of 1-cyclopropyl-7-(4-methyl-piperazinyl)-8-fluoro-quinolones, antibacterial activity increases according to the nature of the substituent in position 5, in the following order:

$R_2N < RH < SH < RO < RNH < Br\ F \leq HO \leq Cl < NH_2$

2.6. Position 6

The nature of the substituent from this position influences the inhibition activity of DNA gyrase and cell penetration.

In this position the following substituents have been introduced: H, F, Cl, Br, CH_3, NO_2, NH_2 [32, 5, 7, 34, 29, 4, 5].

The introduction of a fluorine atom in this position has lead to a spectacular increase of the antibacterial activity, compared to unsubstituted compound (R_6 = H) (activity of norfloxacin against *E. coli* R_6 = F, is 16 times higher than the nonfluorinated compound in position 6) (Table 6).

Regarding the importance of the presence of fluorine atom in position 6 of the quinolone, other authors (Ledoussant et al. 1992) have reported that this is essential for the activity of the quinolone compounds.

R_6	Minimum inhibitory concentration (μg / ml)			Reference
	S. aureus	*E. coli*	*P. aeruginosa*	
H	12.50	0.78	3.13	(Koga et al. 1980)
F: Norfloxacina	0.39	0.05	0.39	(Koga et al. 1980)
Cl	1.56	0.20	3.13	(Koga et al. 1980)
Br	3.13	0.39	1.50	(Koga et al. 1980)
CH_3	3.13	0.39	6.25	(Koga et al. 1980)
SCH_3	25.00	0.78	12.50	(Koga et al. 1980)
$COCH_3$	100.00	100.00	100.00	(Koga et al. 1980)
CN	12.50	0.39	6.25	(Koga et al. 1980)
NO_2	25.00	0.78	12.50	(Koga et al. 1980)

Table 4. The "in vitro" antibacterial activity of 6 substituted quinolones

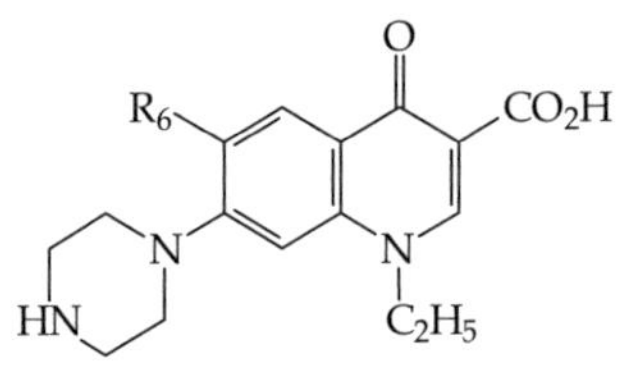

Figure 11. Substituted quinolones.

There have been synthesized compounds containing an amino group at position 6 [3-5]. A direct comparison between 6-amino-quinolones and 6-fluoro-quinolones shows a decrease of antimicrobial activity of 6-amino-quinolones of about 28–300 times (Table 7). The antimicrobial activity of 6-amino-quinolones can be improved by optimizing the chemical structure through the introduction of various substituents in other positions of the quinolones core.

	R_1	**R_5**	**R_7**	**R_8**	**Minimum inhibitory concentration (μg/ml)**			**Reference**
					S. aureus	*E. coli*	*P. aeruginosa*	
1 a	-c-C_3H_5	H	Piperazinyl	H	0.25	64.00	2.00	(Cecheti et al. 1995)
2 a	-c-C_3H5 *ciprofloxacin*	H	Piperazinyl	H	0.12	0.03	0.06	(Cecheti et al. 1995)
1 b	-c-C_3H_5	H	4-Methyl-piperazinil	H	0.25	2.00	4.00	(Cecheti et al. 1995)
1 c	-c-C_3H_5	H	Tiomorpholinyl	F	0.12	0.25	4.00	(Cecheti et al. 1995)
1 d	-c-C_3H_5	NH_2	4-Methyl-piperazinyl	H	128	16	128	(Cecheti et al. 1995)
1 e	-c-C_3H_5	NH_2	4-Methyl-piperazinyl	F	2	0.03	4	(Cecheti et al. 1995)
1 f	-c-C_3H_5	H	4-Methyl-piperazinyl	F	4	1	2	(Cecheti et al. 1995)
1 g	t-Bu	H	4-Methyl-piperazinyl	H	2	0.06	2	(Cecheti et al. 1995)
1 h	4-FC_6H_4	H	4-Methyl-piperazinyl	H	8	0.12	8	(Cecheti et al. 1995)

Table 5. The "in vitro" antibacterial activity of 6-amino-quinolones.

http://dx.doi.org/10.5772/60948

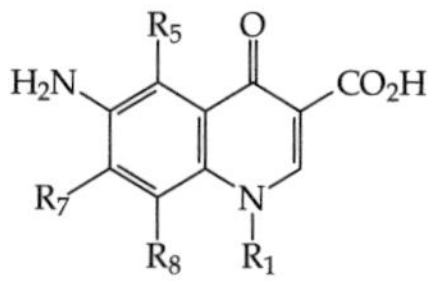

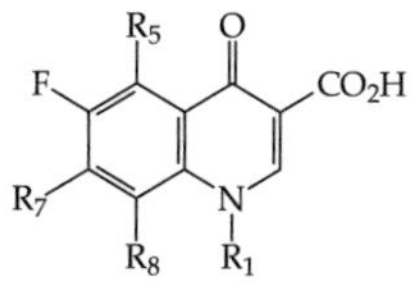

Figure 12. Amino-quinolones and 6-fluoro-quinolones.

2.7. Position 7

Modifications in position 7 have been the most intensively studied; studies have shown that the nature of the substituent from this position has a great influence on the biological potential, antibacterial spectrum, solubility, and on the pharmacokinetics (bioavailability). Research has been focused in the following areas: introduction of piperazinyl, mono or disubstituted piperazinyl, morpholinyl or thiomorpholinyl, pyrrolidinyl, piperidinyl, azetidinyl, bicyclic heterocycles, 4-pyridinyl.

Influence of the nature of the substituent in position 7 on the antibacterial activity is closely related to the nature of the substituents from the other positions of the quinolones core, especially the nature of the substituents at the nitrogen in position 1.

For *1-ethyl-6-fluoro-7-substituted-4-oxo-1,4-dihydro-quinoline-3-carboxylic acid* (Table 6), it was observed that the best influence on antimicrobial activity is the introduction of a piperazinyl group (norfloxacin). Introducing the piperazinyl group in position 7 of the quinolone ring leads to a product with a higher antibacterial potential. The antibacterial spectrum of norfloxacin includes both gram positive and gram negative bacteria, in particular more strains of *P. aeruginosa*.

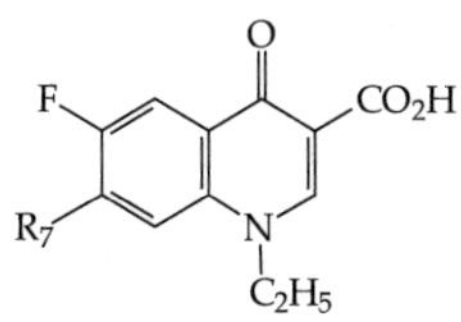

Figure 13. Ethyl-7-substituted-quinolones.

R_7	Minimum inhibitory concentration (μg/ml)			Reference
	S. aureus	*E. coli*	*P. aeruginosa*	
Chlor	12.50	1.56	100.00	(Koga et al.1980)
Methyl	6.25	0.39	5000	(Koga et al.1980)
Amino	100.00	3.13	100.00	(Koga et al.1980)

R_7	Minimum inhibitory concentration (μg/ml)			Reference
	S. aureus	*E. coli*	*P. aeruginosa*	
Methylamino	12.50	3.10	100.00	(Koga et al.1980)
Dimethylamino	0.78	0.39	50.00	(Koga et al.1980)
$S(CH_2)_2NH_2$	25.00	0.80	3.10	(Chu & Fernandes 1991)
Piperazinyl (norfloxacin)	039	0.05	0.39	(Koga et al.1980)
4-Methyl-piperazinyl	0.39	0.10	1.56	(Koga et al.1980)
4-Allyl-piperazinyl	0.39	0.39	6.25	(Koga et al.1980)
4-Benzyl-piperazinyl	0.39	0.79	50.00	(Koga et al.1980)
4- (4-Nitro-benzyl) -piperazinyl	1.56	6.25	100.00	(Koga et al.1980)
4- (4-Amino-benzyl) -piperazinyl	0.39	0.39	12.50	(Koga et al.1980)
4-Benzoyl-piperazinyl	1.56	3.13	25.00	(Koga et al.1980)
4- (2-Hydroxyethyl) piperazinyl	0.78	0.10	6.25	(Koga et al.1980)
3- (Hydroxymethyl) piperazinyl	8.00	2.00	64.00	(Ziegler et al. 1990)
3-Fluoromethyl-piperazinyl	0.12	0.12	32.00	(Ziegler et al. 1990)
3-Difluoromethyl-piperazinyl	0.12	0.50	32.00	(Ziegler et al. 1990)
Morpholinyl	0.78	0.20	12.50	(Koga et al.1980)
Thiomorpholinyl	0.06	1.60	12.50	(Chu & Fernandes 1991)
1-Piperidinyl	0.78	1.56	50.00	(Koga et al.1980)
4-Hydroxy-piperidinyl	0.39	0.39	6.25	(Koga et al.1980)
4-Dimethylamino-piperidinyl	0.39	0.10	3.13	(Koga et al.1980)
Pyrrolidinyl	0.20	0.39	12.50	(Koga et al.1980)
Pyrrolidyl	0.40	1.60	12.50	(Chu & Fernandes 1991)
Thiazolidinyl	0.20	0.20	3.10	(Chu & Fernandes 1991)
1-Imidazolyl	0.25	1.56	12.50	(Toshio et al. 1987)
1-Pyrazolyl	6.25	12.50	25.00	(Toshio et al. 1987)
1-Pyrrolyl	0.39	3.13	12.50	(Toshio et al. 1987)
1,2,4-Triazol-4-yl	25.00	25.00	25.00	(Toshio et al. 1987)
3-Amino-3-methyl-1-azetidinyl	0.50	0.50	2.00	(Toshio et al. 1987)

Table 6. The "in vitro" antibacterial activity of 1-ethyl-7-substituted-quinolones.

For *1-cycloprpyl-6-fluoro-7-substituted-4-oxo-1,4-dihydro-quinoline-3-carboxylic acid* (Table 7) it was observed:

http://dx.doi.org/10.5772/60948

- Introducing a piperazinyl moiety (ciprofloxacin) yields a compound with a higher antibacterial potential; a similar antibacterial activity is obtained in the case where R_7 is 3-methyl-piperazinyl (Compound 1B);
- Introducing the pyrrolidinyl moiety (4A-4E compounds) gives a good bacterial activity on the entire bacterial spectrum, especially in the case of compound 4A where R_7 = 3-amino-pyrrolidinyl;
- Introducing an azetidinyl moiety (Compound 8A) leads to an approximately twofold increase in activity against gram positive bacteria compared to ciprofloxacin; activity against gram negative microorganisms is 4-15 times lower. Introduction of a substituent on the azetidinyl moiety offers compounds with increased activity in the following order: 8I(aminomethyl) ≈ 8J(thia) < 8D(ethylamino) < 8E(dimethylamino) < 8C(methylamino) < 8B(amino). For the 7-(3,3-di-azetidinyl)-quinolone, antibacterial activity increases in the following order: 8K (aminomethyl) ≈ 8L (ethylaminomethyl) < 8H (dimethylamino) < 8C (methylamino) < 8F (amino). In conclusion, the activity "in vitro" of the compounds 8B and 8F increases on the entire bacterial spectrum and can be compared with that of ciprofloxacin. For compounds where R_7 are 3-amino-2-methyl-azetidinyl (compounds 9A–9H), the effect given by the stereochemistry of the substituents in the azetidinyl moiety has been studied. The activity "in vitro" of the compound trans-7-(3-amino-2-methyl-azetidinyl) quinolone 9A can be compared favorably with the activity of 3-monosubstituted-azetidinyl, 3,3-disubstituted-azetidinyl and ciprofloxacin.

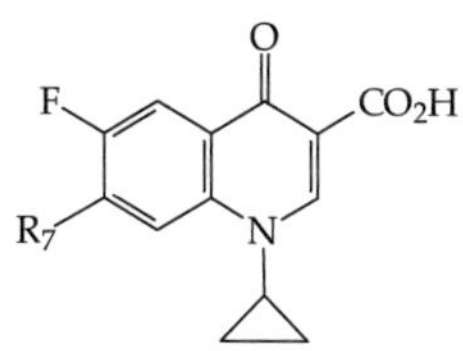

Figure 14. Cyclopropyl-7-substituted-quinolones.

Comp.	R_7	Minimum inhibitory concentration (μg/ml)			Reference
		S. aureus	*E. coli*	*P. aeruginosa*	
1A	Piperazinyl (ciprofloxacin)	0.13	0.03	0.13	(Bouzard et al. 1989)
1B	3-Methyl-piperazinyl	0.12	0.015	0.25	(Ziegler et al. 1990)
1C	3-Fluoromethyl-piperazinyl	0.12	0.06	2.00	
2A	Morpholinyl	0.05	0.20	1.56	(Kazico et al. 1993)
2B	3-Aminomethyl-morpholinyl	0.20	0.20	1.56	

Comp.	R_7	Minimum inhibitory concentration (μg/ml)			Reference
		S. aureus	*E. coli*	*P. aeruginosa*	
3A	Homopiperazinyl	0.25	0.03	1.00	(Ziegler et al. 1990)
3B	3-Hydroxy-homopiperazinyl	4.00	0.25	2.00	
3C	3-Fluoro-homopiperazinyl	0.25	0.03	2.00	
4A	3-Amino-pyrrolidinyl	0.025	0.025	0.1-0.2	(Domagala et al.1993)
4B	3-Aminomethyl-pyrrolidinyl	0.006	0.05	0.80	
4C	3-Methylamino-pyrrolidinyl	0.025	0.10	0.80	
4D	3-Thia-pyrrolidinyl	0.013	0.20	1.6	
4E	3-Aminomethyl-3-methyl-pyrrolidinyl	0013	0.20	0.80	
5	3-Hydroxy-pyrrolidinyl	<0.015	<0.015	0.125	(Petersen & Grohe 1992)
6	3-Oxo-pyrrolidinyl	1.56	6.20	100.00	(Cooper et al. 1992)
7A	3-Amino-4-trans-cyclopropyl-pyrrolidinyl	<0.025	0.05	0.80	(Bush et al. 1993)
7B	3-Amino-4-trans-(trans-2-CO_2Et)-cyclopropyl- pyrrolidinyl	0.20	0.20	3.10	
8A	Azetidinyl	0.06	0.12	2.00	(Frigola et al. 1993)
8B	3-Amino-azetidinyl	0.25	0.03	0.25	
8C	3-Methylamino-azetidinyl	0.25	0.03	0.50	
8D	3-Ethylamino-azetidinyl	0.25	0.06	2.00	
8E	3-Dimethylamino-azetidinyl	0.12	0.06	2.00	
8F	3-Methyl-3-amino-azetidinyl	0.12	0.06	0.50	
8G	3-Methylamino-3-methyl-azetidinyl	0.25	0.06	2.00	
8H	3-Dimethylamino-3-methyl-azetidinyl	0.25	0.25	4.00	
8I	3-Aminoethyl-azetidinyl	0.50	0.12	1.00	
8J	3-Thia-azetidinyl	0.50	0.25	4.00	
8K	3-Aminomethyl-3-methyl-azetidinyl	0.25	0.12	1.00	
8L	3-Thia-3-methyl-azetidinyl	0.25	0.12	4.00	
9	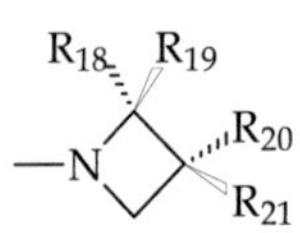				(Frigola et al. 1994)
	R_{18} **R_{19}** **R_{20}** **R_{21}**				

http://dx.doi.org/10.5772/60948

Comp.	R_7				Minimum inhibitory concentration (μg/ml)			Reference
					S. aureus	*E. coli*	*P. aeruginosa*	
9A	CH_3	H	H	NH_2	0,12.	0.03	0.25	
9B	CH_3	H	NH_2	H	0.12	0.06	0.50	
9C	C_2H_5	H	NH_2	H	0.25	0.12	2.00	
9D	H	CH_3	NH_2	CH_3	0.25	0.06	2.00	
9E	H	CH_3	$NHCH_3$	H	0.12	0.06	0.50	
9F	H	CH_3	$N(CH_3)_2$	H	0.25	0.50	4.00	
9G	H	CH_3	CH_2NH_2	H	0.25	0.12	2.00	
9H	H	CH_3	$CH_2NHC_2H_5$	H	0.25	0.12	4.00	

Table 7. The "in vitro" antibacterial activity of 1-cyclopropyl-7-substituted-quinolones.

For *1-(p-fluorophenyl)-7-substituted-quinolones* (Table 8), it is observed that the introduction of substituents: 3-methyl-piperazinyl (4), 4-amino-piperazinyl (8), 3 amino-pyrrolidinyl) (17), and 3-methyl-2-amino-pyrrolidinyl (20) has the effect of extending of the antibacterial spectrum on both gram positive and gram negative bacteria, while introducing morpholinyl groups (10), thiomorpholinyl (11), 4-hydroxy-piperidinyl (13), pyrrolidinyl (15), 3-hydroxy-pyrrolidinyl (compound 16) leads to the increase of antibacterial activity against gram positive bacteria, comparable with the antibacterial activity of the sarafloxacin and difloxacin. It should be noted that the introduction of the methyl group in position 5 of 3-amino-pyrrolidinyl substituent (compound 17) leads to obtaining a compound (20) with a high solubility in water and with excellent efficacy in oral administration.

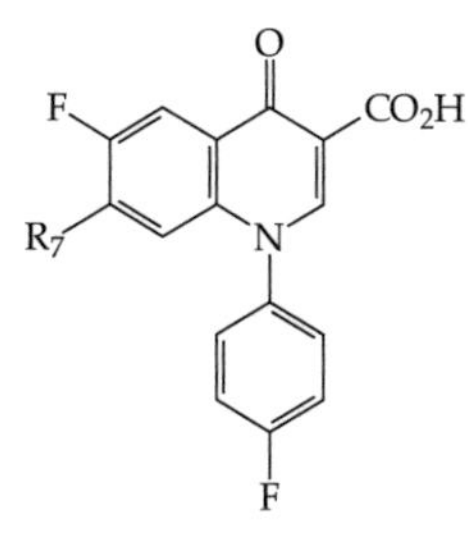

Figure 15. *p*-Fluorophenyl)-7-substituted-quinolones.

Structural changes were focused on replacing the nitrogen atom of the heterocyclic substituent with a sp^2 or sp^3 hybridized carbon atom. All new compounds have a high activity both "in vitro" and "in vivo". The potential of these compounds is relatively dependent on the size of the ring and the hybridization of the carbon atom through which it connects with the quinolone. 1-Piperazino moiety can be substituted with 4-piperidinyl (compound 1, Table 9) with

	R_7	Minimum inhibitory concentration (μg/ml)			Reference
		S. aureus	*E. coli*	*P. aeruginosa*	
1	Piperazinyl (sarafloxacina)	0.20	0.05	0.39	(Chu et al. 1985)
2	4-Methyl-piperazinyl (difloxacin)	0.20	0.20	1.56	(Chu et al. 1985)
3	4-Butyl-piperazinyl	0.78	1.56	12.50	(Chu et al. 1985)
4	3-Methyl-piperazinyl	0.20	<0.05	0.78	(Chu & Fernandes 1991)
5	3,5-Dimethyl-piperazinyl	0.39	<0.05	1.56	(Chu & Fernandes 1991)
6	3-Fluoromethyl-piperazinyl	0.25	0.25	2.00	(Domagala et al. 1988)
7	3-Oxo-piperazinyl	0.20	0.20	1.56	(Chu et al. 1985)
8	4-Amino-piperazinyl	0.39	0.20	0.78	(Chu & Fernandes 1991)
9	Homopiperazinyl	0.79	0.20	1.56	(Chu et al. 1985)
10	Morpholinyl	0.10	0.39	3.10	(Chu et al. 1985)
11	Thiomorpholinyl	0.05	0.78	3.10	(Chu et al. 1985)
12	Piperidinyl	0.20	1.56	6.20	(Chu et al. 1985)
13	4-Hydroxy-piperidinyl	0.10	0.39	6.20	(Chu et al. 1985)
14	4-Dimethylamino-piperidinyl	0.39	0.73	3.10	(Chu et al. 1985)
15	Pyrrolidinyl	0.10	0.78	1.56	(Chu et al. 1985)
16	3-Hydroxy-pyrrolidinyl	0.10	0.20	3.10	(Chu et al. 1985)
17	3-Amino-pyrrolidinyl	0.10	<0.05	0.78	(Chu & Fernandes 1991)
18	3-Methylamino-pyrrolidinyl	0.20	<0.05	1.56	(Chu & Fernandes 1991)
19	3-Dimethylamino-pyrrolidinyl	0.78	<0.05	6.25	(Chu & Fernandes 1991)
20	3-Methyl-3-amino-pyrrolidinyl	0.05	0.02	0.78	(Rosen et al. 1988)
21	Trans (3-amino-2-methyl) -azetidinyl	0.25	0.12	1.00	(Domagala et al. 1988)
22	3-Amino-3-methyl-azetidinyl	0.12	0.12	2.00	(Domagala et al. 1988)

6-Fluoro-1,4-dihydro-4-oxo-quinoline-3-carboxylic acids substituted in position 7 with bioisosteric non-basic groups.

Table 8. The "in vitro" antibacterial activity of 1-(*p*-fluorophenyl)-7-substituted-quinolones.

4-(1,2,3,6-tetrahydropyridinyl) (compound 2), while the 3-amino-pyrrolidinyl moiety can be substituted with 3-amino-cyclopentanyl (compound 3). For the compounds 1 and 2, the nature of isosteric atom that replaces the nitrogen atom in position 1 of the piperazinyl moiety influences the antimicrobial activity "in vitro" as follows: while this sp^2 hybridized atom (through which connects the quinolone nucleus) leads to compounds (2) with activity comparable to ciprofloxacin, the presence of carbon sp^3 leads to decreased activity "in vitro" of about 4–12 times. Replacement of the 3-amino-1-pyrrolidinyl (compound B) with 3-amino-1-

http://dx.doi.org/10.5772/60948

cyclopentanyl (compound 3) results in a decrease in antimicrobial activity. In general, the piperazinyl moiety in position 7 has a favorable influence at the "in vitro" activity, but 7-substituted piperazinyl quinolones do not have a good availability.

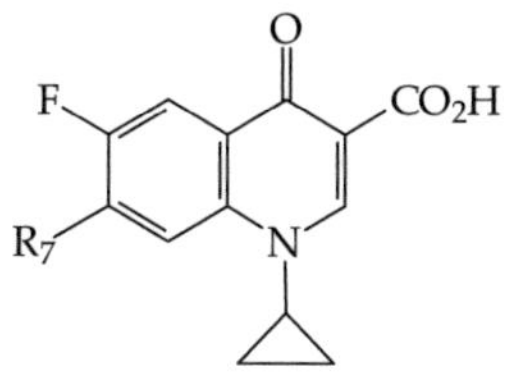

Figure 16. Cyclopropyl-quinolones substituted in position 7 with bioisosteric non-basic groups.

Compound	R_7	Minimum inhibitory concentration (µg / ml)			Reference
		S. aureus	*E. coli*	*P. aeruginosa*	
A	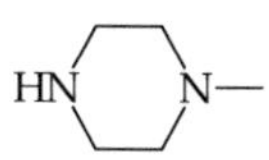	0.13	0.03	0.13	(Bouzard et al. 1989)
1	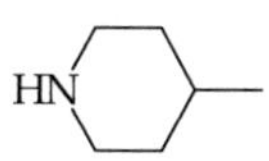	0.80	0.20	1.60	(Laborde et al. 1993)
2	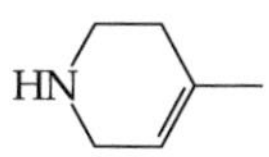	0.10	0.025	0.80	(Laborde et al. 1993)
B	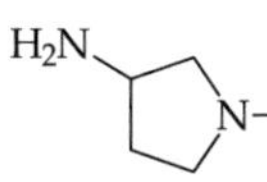	0.025	0.025	0.20	(Laborde et al. 1993)
3	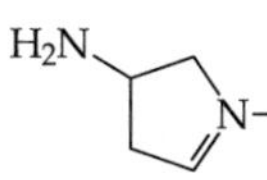	0.10	0.10	0.80	(Laborde et al. 1993)

Table 9. The "in vitro" antibacterial activity of 1-cyclopropyl-quinolones substituted in position 7 with bioisosteric non-basic groups.

2.8. Position 8

The most famous modifications of the 8 position of the quinolone are X = CH or N (naphthyridines). However, compact and lipophilic groups: X = CR_8, where R_8 = fluorine [16, 17, 25, 54], trifluoromethyl [52] and methoxy [22, 55] have gained ground due to the positive influence they have on the antibacterial activity.

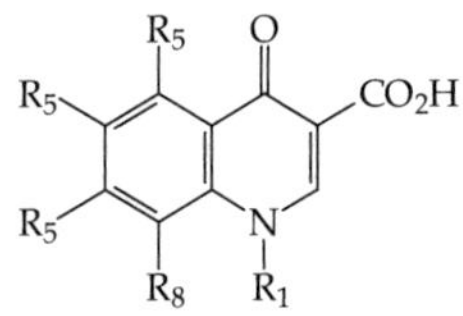

R_8 = F, Cl, OCH_3 > H, CF_3 > methyl, vinyl, propargyl

Figure 17. Influence of the nature of the substituent at 8 position on the antimicrobial activity.

In general, the introduction of a fluorine atom in 8 position leads to increased antibacterial activity against gram negative microorganisms, while introducing the methoxy group increase the activity only against the gram positive bacteria.

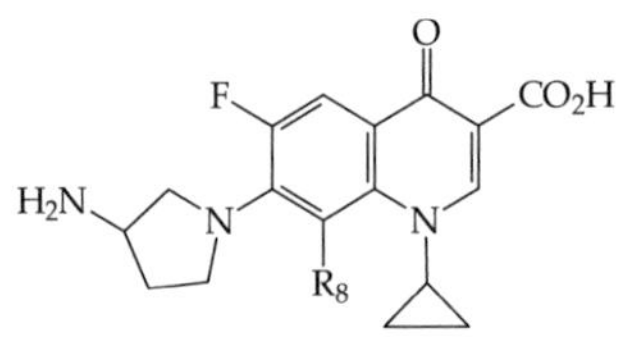

Figure 18. Cyclopropyl-8-substituted quinolones.

R_8	Minimum inhibitory concentration (μG / ML) geometric mean	
	Gram (-)organisms	Gram (+)organisms
H	0.09	0.14
F	0.04	0.03
OMe	0.07	0.03
Cl	0.03	0.04
NO_2	0.46	0.92
NH_2	0.53	0.06
CF_3	0.20	0.20
SMe	0.20	0.06

Table 10. The "in vitro" antibacterial activity 8 substituted quinolones.

The compounds containing a chlorine atom in 8 position [30, 25, 17] are very active, as well as analogs containing fluorine or methoxy moiety [22, 55]. The introduction of bulky substituents, e.g., ethyl, reduces the antibacterial activity against gram negative (if a comparison with 8-methoxy-quinolones is made). Quinolones having a halogen atom, fluorine or chlorine in 8

http://dx.doi.org/10.5772/60948

position, show the phototoxicity; the introduction of trifluoromethyl group [52] leads to reduced cytotoxicity. Alkylation of carbon in position 8 is tolerated, especially if the substituent is lipophilic and has a small volume. Thus the introduction of the methyl group [4, 5] leads to compounds with modest antibacterial activity. Instead, amino, nitro, hydroxy substituents lead to loss of antibacterial activity (Dax 1997).

3. New compounds: synthesis, structure and antimicrobial activity

3.1. Structure of the new compounds

A series of 4-oxo-1,4-dihydro-quinoline-3-carboxylic acids was synthesized. (Figure 19) (Table 11). Their structure has been determined and confirmed by the following physicochemical methods: elemental analysis, IR spectral analysis, H-NMR, C-NMR, UV, thin layer chromatography.

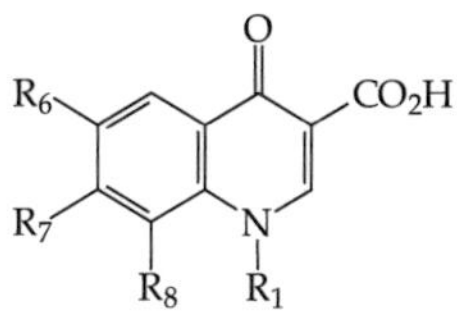

Figure 19. Structure of 4-oxo-1,4-dihydro-quinoline-3-carboxylic acids.

Quinolones	R_1	R_6	R_7	R_8	m.p. (°C)	Reference
FPQ 24 $C_{18}H_{21}FN_2O_3$	Ethyl	F	3-Methyl-piperidin-1-yl	H	189.4	Pintilie et al. (2009b)
FPQ 30 $C_{18}H_{20}ClFN_2O_3$	Ethyl	F	3-Methyl-piperidin-1-yl	Cl	163-165.3	Pintilie et al. (2014a)
FPQ 32 $C_{17}H_{19}FN_2O_3$	Ethyl	F	Piperidin-1-yl	H	202.4-204.4	Pintilie & Nita (2011a)
FPQ 33 $C_{17}H_{18}ClFN_2O_3$	Ethyl	F	Piperidin-1-yl	Cl	186-191.2	Pintilie & Nita (2011a)
Q 83 $C_{18}H_{21}FN_2O_3$	Ethyl	F	4-Methyl-piperidin-1-yl	H	235-237	Pintilie et al. (2003b)
Q 85 $C_{18}H_{20}ClFN_2O_3$	Ethyl	F	4-Methyl-piperidin-1-yl	Cl	201-202.5	Pintilie et al. (2003b)
FPQ 35 $C_{16}H_{17}FN_2O_3$	Ethyl	F	Pyrrolidin-1-yl	H	336.6-337.9	Pintilie & Nita (2011a)
FPQ 36	Ethyl	F	Pyrrolidin-1-yl	Cl	214.5-217.8	Pintilie & Nita (2011a)

Quinolones	R1	R6	R7	R8	m.p. (°C)	Reference
$C_{16}H_{16}ClFN_2O_3$						
FPQ 25 $C_{16}H_{17}FN_2O_4$	Ethyl	F	Morpholin-1-yl	H	257.4-258.7	Pintilie et al. (2009b)
FPQ 28 $C_{16}H_{16}ClFN_2O_4$	Ethyl	F	Morpholin-1-yl	Cl	244.6-244	Pintilie et al. (2014a)
NF $C_{16}H_{18}FN_3O_3$	Ethyl	F	Piperazin-1-yl	H	218-220	Pintilie et al. (2014b)
AcNF $C_{18}H_{20}FN_3O_4$	Ethyl	F	4-Acetyl-piperazin-1-yl	H	297.8-299.9	Pintilie et al. (2014b)
AcFPQ 50 $C_{18}H_{19}ClFN_3O_4$	Ethyl	F	4-Acetyl-piperazin-1-yl	Cl	255.7-258.2	Pintilie et al. (2014b)
FPQ 50 $C_{16}H_{17}ClFN_3O_3$	Ethyl	F	Piprazin-1-yl	Cl	227-230	Pintilie et al. (2014b)
PF $C_{17}H_{20}FN_3O_3$	Ethyl	F	4-Methyl-piperazin-1-yl	H	269.2-272.8	Pintilie et al. (2014b)
FPQ 51 $C_{17}H_{19}ClFN_3O_3$	Ethyl	F	4-Methyl-piperazin-1-yl	Cl	219.6-221	Pintilie et al. (2014b)
FPQ 27 $C_{17}H_{20}FN_2O_3$	Ethyl	F	3-Methyl-piperazin-1-yl	H	177.6-180.6	Pintilie et al. (2014a)
AcFPQ 27 $C_{19}H_{22}FN_3O_4$	Ethyl	F	4-Acetyl-3-methyl-piperazin-1-yl	H	247.5-248.9	Pintilie & Nita (2011a)
AcFPQ29 $C_{19}H_{21}ClFN_3O_4$	Ethyl	F	4-Acetyl-3-methyl-piperazin-1-yl	Cl	262.7-264.8	Pintilie & Nita (2011a)
FPQ29 . HCl $C_{17}H_{29}ClFN_2O_3.HCl$	Ethyl	F	3-Methyl-piperazin-1-yl	Cl	280-283	Pintilie & Nita (2011a)
6ClPQ 24 $C_{18}H_{21}ClN_2O_3$	Ethyl	Cl	3-Methyl-piperidin-1-yl	H	216,4-218,4	Pintilie et al. (2009b)
6ClPQ 30 $C_{18}H_{20}Cl_2N_2O_3$	Ethyl	Cl	3-Methyl-piperidin-1-yl	Cl	190.3-192.2	Pintilie & Nita (2011b)
6ClPQ 32 $C_{17}H_{19}ClN_2O_3$	Ethyl	Cl	Piperidin-1-yl	H	234.6-236.4	Pintilie & Nita (2011b)
6ClPQ 33 $C_{17}H_{18}Cl_2N_2O_3$	Ethyl	Cl	Piperidin-1-yl	Cl	214.6-216.3	Pintilie & Nita (2011b)
PQ 80 $C_{18}H_{21}ClN_2O_3$	Ethyl	Cl	4-Methyl-piperidin-1-yl	H	262.5-264.4	Pintilie & Nita (2011b)
PQ87 $C_{18}H_{20}Cl_2N_2O_3$	Ethyl	Cl	4-Methyl-piperidin-1-yl	Cl	152.3-154.9	Pintilie & Nita (2011b)
6ClPQ 35 $C_{17}H_{18}Cl_2N_2O_3$	Ethyl	Cl	Pyrrolidin-1-yl	H	312.3-315.5	Pintilie & Nita (2011b)

Quinolones	R_1	R_6	R_7	R_8	m.p. (°C)	Reference
6ClPQ 36 $C_{17}H_{18}Cl_2N_2O_3$	Ethyl	Cl	Pyrrolidin-1-yl	Cl	172.4-176.1	Pintilie & Nita (2011b)
6ClPQ 25 $C_{16}H_{17}ClN_2O_4$	Ethyl	Cl	Morpholin-1-yl	H	267,1-269,2	Pintilie et al. (2009b)
6ClPQ 28 $C_{16}H_{16}Cl_2N_2O_4$	Ethyl	Cl	Morpholin-1-yl	Cl	213.9-216.7	Pintilie & Nita (2011b)
NClX $C_{16}H_{18}ClN_3O_3$	Ethyl	Cl	Piperazin-1-yl	H	226.8-228.5	Pintilie et al. (2014b)
AcNClX $C_{18}H_{20}ClN_3O_4$	Ethyl	Cl	4-Acetyl-piperazin-1-yl	H	306-310	Pintilie et al. (2014b)
Ac6ClPQ 50 $C_{18}H_{19}Cl_2N_3O_4$	Ethyl	Cl	4-Acetyl-piperazin-1-yl	Cl	260.1-263.7	Pintilie et al. (2014b)
6ClPQ 50 $C_{16}H_{17}Cl_2N_3O_3$	Ethyl	Cl	Piperazin-1-yl	Cl	228.2-230.4	Pintilie et al. (2014b)
PClX $C_{17}H_{20}ClN_3O_3$	Ethyl	Cl	4-Methyl-piperazin-1-yl	H	253.7-258.2	Pintilie et al. (2014b)
6ClPQ 51 $C_{17}H_{19}Cl_2N_3O_3$	Ethyl	Cl	4-Methyl-piperazin-1-yl	Cl	223.4-226	Pintilie et al. (2014b)
6ClPQ 27 $C_{17}H_{20}ClN_3O_3$	Ethyl	Cl	3-Methyl-piperazin-1-yl	H	170.5-171.4	Pintilie et al. (2009b)
Ac6ClPQ 27 $C_{19}H_{22}ClN_3O_4$	Ethyl	Cl	4-Acetyl-3-methyl-piperazin-1-yl	H	275-276	Pintilie et al. (2014 b)
Ac6ClPQ 29 $C_{19}H_{21}Cl_2N_3O_4$	Ethyl	Cl	4-Acetyl-3-methyl-piperazin-1-yl	Cl	210.3-211.7	Pintilie et al. (2014b)
6ClPQ 29 $C_{17}H_{19}Cl_2N_2O_3$	Ethyl	Cl	3-Methyl-piperazin-1-yl	Cl	278.5-282	Pintilie et al. (2014b)

Table 11. Oxo-1,4-dihydro-quinoline-3-carboxylic acids synthesized.

3.2. Synthesis pathway

The synthesis of the novel quinolones followed a Gould–Jacobs cyclization process (Scheme 1). Appropriate unsubstituted aniline (1) is reacted with diethylethoxy methylene malonate (EMME) to produce the resultant anilinomethylenemalonate. A subsequent thermal process induces Gould–Jacobs cyclization to afford the corresponding 4-hidroxy-quinoline-3-carboxylate ester (2). The following operation is the alkylation of the quinolone, which is usually accomplished by reaction with a suitable alkyl halide or dialkyl sulphates to produce the qinolone-3-carboxylate ester (3). The final manipulation is acid or basic hydrolysis to cleave the ester generating the biologically active free carboxylic acid (4). The biologically active free carboxylic acid (4) was also obtained from the corresponding 4-hidroxy-quinoline-3-carboxylate ester (2) by alkylation with dialkyl sulphates in presence of alkali, for example, the reaction it can conveniently be carried out in aqueous 40% sodium hydroxide solution. The displacement of 7-chloro group with a heterocyclic yielded compounds (5). 8-Chloro-quinoline-3-carboxylic acid (8) was synthesized from 8-unsubstituted quinoline-3-carboxylic acid (5) by chlorination with sulfuryl chloride (when R_7 = 4-methyl-piperazine). When R_7 = 3-methyl-piperazine or piperazine, it is necessary to protect the nitrogen atom from piperazine group. After chlorination and hydrolysis, the final compound (8) is obtained (R_7 = 3-methyl-piperazine, or piperazine).

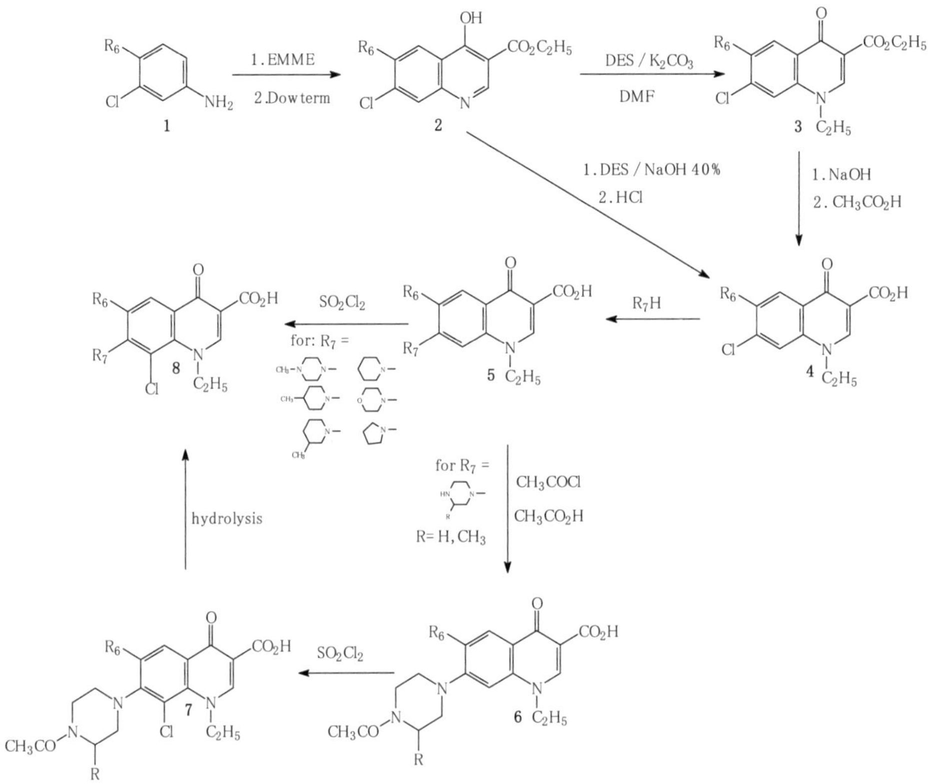

Figure 20. Synthesis of the new quinolones.

3.3. Antibacterial activity of the new compounds

The new compounds were evaluated for "in vitro" activity by determining minimum inhibitory concentration against bacteria *E. coli*, *S. aureus*, and *P. aeruginosa*, by agar dilution method (Buiuc 1998) (NCCLS 2003) (Table 12). After analyzing chemical structure–biological activity relationships, it was observed that the presence of chlorine in 8 position of the quinolones core leads to increased antimicrobial activity for the compounds having piperidinyl, morpholinyl, and pyrrolidinyl moiety in 7-position. For 7-piperazinyl quinolones, the chlorine atom from 8-position leads to decreased activity against all the tested strains.

Quinolone	Minimum inhibitory concentration μg/ml			References
	E. coli (a)	*S. aureus* (b)	*P. aeruginosa* (c)	
FPQ 24	2.00	0.50	32.00	Pintilie et al. 2009b
FPQ 30	0.32	0.125	1.28	Pintilie & Nita 2011a
FPQ 32	1.00	8.00	8.00	Pintilie & Nita 2011a
FPQ 33	0.32	0.32	1.28	Pintilie & Nita 2011a
Q 83	3,12	1,56	6,25	Pintilie et al. 2003b
Q 85	3,12	0,39	6,25	Pintilie et al. 2003b
FPQ 35	31.25	1.953	"/>125	Pintilie & Nita 2011a
FPQ 36	15.625	0.244	15.625	Pintilie & Nita 2011a
FPQ 28	0,125	0,06	8,00	Pintilie et al. (2009b)
NF	<0.08	0.32	0.32	Pintilie et al. 2014 b
FPQ 50	2.00	4.00	16.00	Pintilie et al. 2014 b
PF	<0.08	1.28	1.28	Pintilie et al. 2014 b
FPQ 51	2.00	4.00	32.00	Pintilie et al. 2014 b
FPQ 27	0.125	1.00	1.00	Pintilie & Nita 2011a
FPQ 29	0.30	1.21	4.83	Pintilie & Nita 2011a
6ClPQ 24	8,00	2,00	"/>128	Pintilie et al. (2009b)
6ClPQ 30	8.00	2.56	2.56	Pintilie & Nita 2011b
6ClPQ 33	2.56	2.56	2.56	Pintilie & Nita 2011b
6ClPQ 36	2.56	2.56	2.56	Pintilie & Nita 2011b
6ClPQ 28	1.28	1.28	64	Pintilie & Nita 2011b
NClX	0.32	1.28	5.12	Pintilie et al. 2014 b
6ClPQ 50	2.00	8.00	32.00	Pintilie et al. 2014 b
PClX	0.32	1.28	5.12	Pintilie et al. 2014 b
6ClPQ 51	3.906	15.625	62.5	Pintilie et al. 2014 b

a. *E. coli ATCC 8739*, b. *S. aureus ATCC 6538*, c. *P. aeruginosa ATCC 9027*

Table 12. "In vitro" antibacterial activity of the new quinolones.

3.4. Antibacterial activity of the new compounds against methicillin-resistant *S. aureus*

Some of the new quinolones, which showed a good activity, have been tested against 30 strains of methicillin-resistant *S. aureus* isolated in the Microbiology Laboratory of INBI Prof. "Dr. Matei Bals" during 2012. The minimum inhibitory concentration (MIC) of the isolates has been determined by agar plate Mueller Hinton (bioMerieux) dilution method using the reference strain *S. aureus* ATCC 29213. The 30 strains of isolated have been also tested for susceptibility to ciprofloxacin, levofloxacin, and imipenem by Etest method.

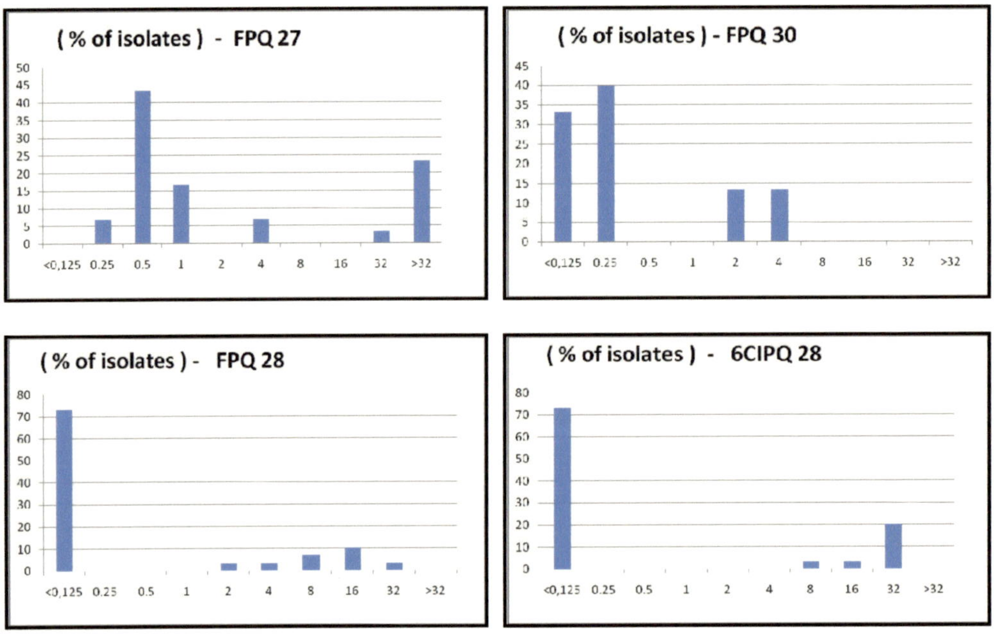

Figure 21. MIC histograms of 4 quinolones against 30 strains of methicillin-resistant *S. aureus*.

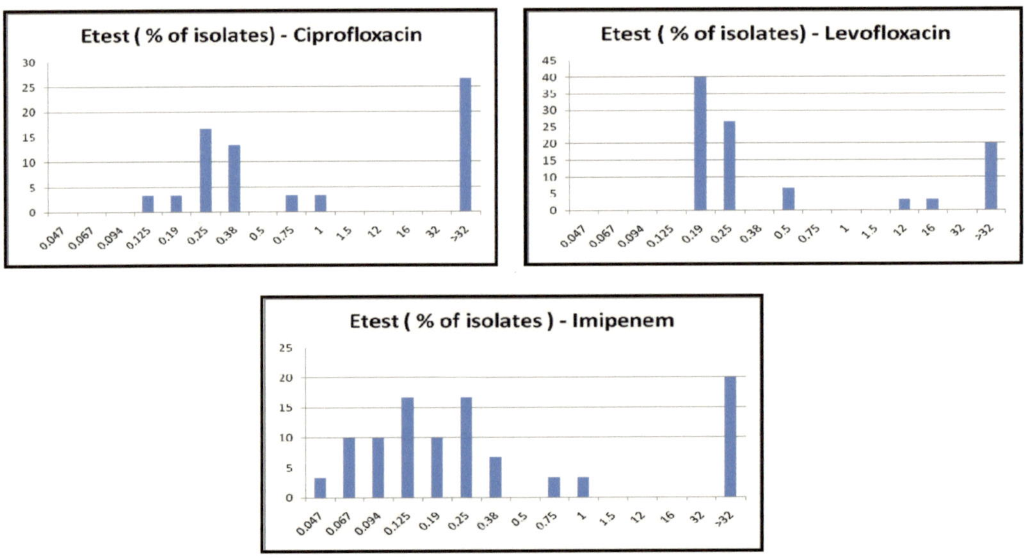

Figure 22. MIC histograms of ciprofloxacin, levofloxacin, imipenem against 30 strains of methicillin-resistant *S. aureus*, determined by Etest method.

Base on the "in vitro" studies, the quinolone FPQ-30 appears to be a promising compound; all strains isolates were inhibited at a concentration of 8 μg/ml (Figure 21).

4. Conclusion

In conclusion, we have synthesized new quinolone compounds and we have investigated their activity against multidrug-resistant gram positive microorganisms. Of the four compounds, FPQ-30 (Figure 23, 24) showed the best activity; all strains isolates were inhibited at a concentration of 8 μg/ml. The results of the present study indicate the quinolone FPQ-30 appears to be a promising compound.

Its structure has been determined and confirmed by the following physicochemical methods: elemental analysis, IR spectral analysis, H-NMR, C-NMR, UV (Figure 25) and thin layer chromatography.

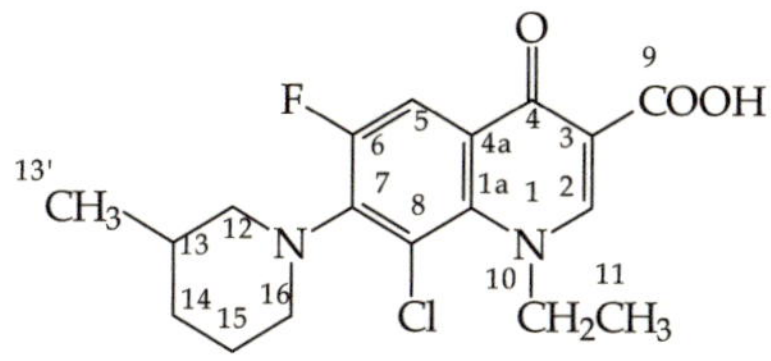

^{1}H-NMR(dmso-d6, δ ppm, J Hz, T = 333K): 8.88(s, 1H, H-2); 7.93(d, 1H, H-5, ^3J(F-H^5) = 13.4 Hz); 4.81(q, 2H, H-10, 7.1); 3.28(m, 2H, H-16, H-12); 3.11(dd, 1H, H-12, 10.7, 12.1); 2.81(td, 1H, H-16, 12.1, 2.9); 1.58 ÷ 1.86(m, H, H-13, 2H-14, 1H-15); 1.39(t, 3H, H-11, 7.1); 1.13(qd, 1H, H-15, 10.8, 4.1); 0.88(d, 3H, H-13, 6.4).

^{13}C-NMR(dmso-d6, δ ppm): 175.89(d, C-4, ^4J(F-C^4) = 2.8 Hz); 167.30(C-9); 155.83(d, C-6, J(F-C^6) = 251.1 Hz); 152.45(C-2); 144.37(d, C-7, ^2J(F-C^7) = 14.3 Hz); 136.46(C-1a); 122.95(d, C-4a, ^3J(F-C^{4a}) = 7.1 Hz); 118.93(C-8); 110.79(d, C-5, ^2J(F-C^5) = 23.4 Hz); 107.67(C-3); 58.70 (d, C-12, ^4J(F-C^{12}) = 4.6 Hz); 53.06(C-10); 51.57(d, C-16, ^4J(F-C^{16}) = 4.6 Hz); 32.05(C-15); 31.17(C-13); 25.39(C-14); 18.82(C-13);15.73(C-11).

FT-IR(solid in ATR, ν/cm): 3059m; 2947w; 2925m; 2867w; 2845m; 1719vs; 1616s; 1558s; 1531m; 1489m; 1437vs; 1381m; 1319m; 1294m; 1250m; 1229m; 1208m; 1189m; 1125w; 1101m; 1081m; 1040m; 996w; 968w; 926m; 887m; 857w; 838w; 8.05m; 741w.

Figure 23. Ethyl-6-fluoro-7-(4-methyl-piperidinyl)-8-chloro- Optimized molecular structure of FPQ 30

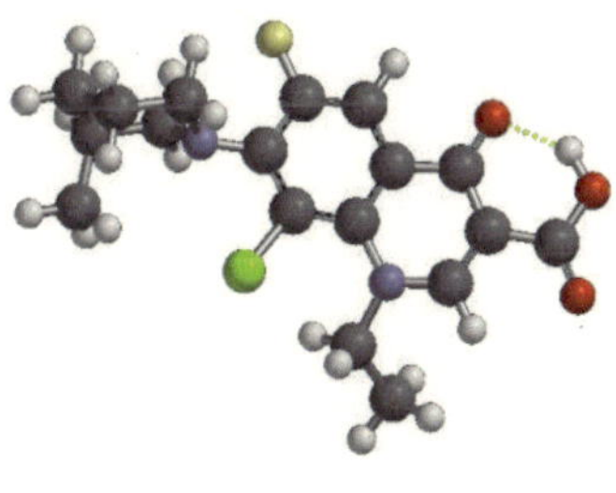

Figure 24. dihydro-4-oxo-quinoline-3-carboxylic acid (FPQ 30) with Spartan 14 Software

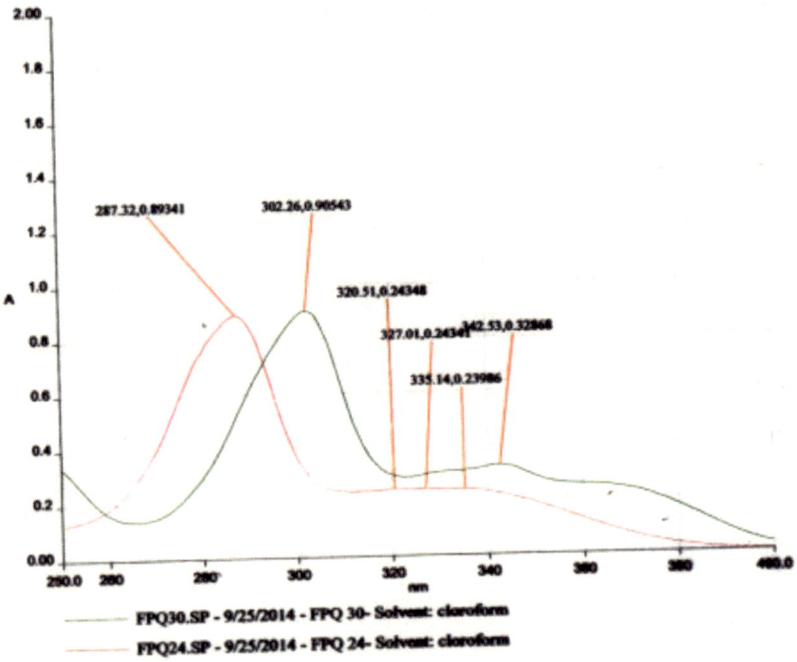

Figure 25. UV absorption spectrum of FPQ-24 and FPQ-30

UV absorption spectra study was carried out using solutions with oncentration of 10 mg/ml in chloroform. Interpretation of the UV absorption spectrum has been made in comparison with that of the quinolone compound: 1-ethyl-6-fluoro-7-(3-methyl-piperidin-1-yl)-1,4-dihydro-4-oxo-quinoline-3-carboxylic acid (FPQ 24), namely:

- The presence of the quinolone nucleus determines in chloroform the appearance of electronic transitions in the field of 260–310 nm and 320–350 nm.
- The introduction of chlorine atom in 8 position produces a batocroma displacement of the entire spectrum.

Author details

Pintilie Lucia*

Address all correspondence to: lucia.pintilie@gmail.com

National Institute for Chemical-Pharmaceutical Research & Development–Bucharest, Romania

References

[1] Bouzard D, DiCesare P, Essiz M, Jacquet JP, Remuzon P, Weber A, Oki T, Masuyoshi M. Fluoronaphthyridines and quinolones as antibacterial agents. 1. Synthesis and structure-activity relationship of new 1-substituted derivatives. J Med Chem 1989;32(3):537–42, ISSN-0022-2623.

[2] Bush AR, Domagala JM, Laborde E, Sesnie JC. Synthesis and antimicrobial evaluation of a series of 7-[3-amino (or aminomethyl)-4-aryl (or cyclopropyl)-1-pyrrolidinyl]-4-quinolone and -1,8-naphthyridone-3-carboxylic acids. J Med Chem 1993;36(26):4139–59, ISSN-0022-2623.

[3] Cecchetti V, Clementi S, Cruciani G, Fravolini A, Pagella PG, Savino A, Tabarini O. 6-Aminoquinolones: a new class of quinolone antibacterials? J Med Chem 1995;38(6): 973–82, ISSN-0022-2623.

[4] Cechetti V, Fravolini A, Lorenzini MC, Tabarrini O, Terni P, Xin T. Studies on 6-Aminoquinolones: synthesis and antibacterial evaluation of 6-Amino-8-methylquinolones. J Med Chem 1996a;39(2):436–45, ISSN-0022-2623.

[5] Cechetti V, Fravolini A., Palumbo M, Sissi C, Tabarrini O, Terni P, Xin, T. Potent 6-desfluoro-8-methylquinolones as new lead compounds in antibacterial chemotherapy. J Med Chem 1996b:39(25):4952–7, ISSN-0022-2623.

[6] Cechetti V, Filipponi E, Fravolini A, Tabarrini O, Bonelli D, Clementi M, Cruciani G, Clementi S. Chemometric methodologies in a quantitative structure–activity relationship study: the antibacterial activity of 6-aminoquinolones. J Med Chem 1997;40(11):1698–706, ISSN-0022-2623.

[7] Chu DTW, Fernandes P, Claiborne AK, Pihuleac E, Norden CW, Maleczka JRE, Pernet AG. Synthesis and structure-activity relationships of novel arylfluoroquinolone antibacterial agents. J Med Chem 1985;28(12):1558–64, ISSN-0022-2623.

[8] Chu DTW, Fernandes PB, Maleczka Jr RE, Nordeen CW, Pernet AG. Synthesis and structure-activity relationship of 1-aryl-6,8-difluoroquinolone antibacterial agents. J Med Chem 1987;30(3):504–9, ISSN-0022-2623.

[9] Chu DTW, Fernandes P. Recent developments in the field of quinolone antibacterial agents. In: Advances in Drug Research, 1991, Vol. 21, Bernard Testa, pp.39–144, Academic Press, ISBN 0-12-013321-0, London; San Diego; New York.

[10] Cooper CS, Klock PL, Chu DTW, Fernandes PB. The synthesis and antibacterial activities of quinolones containing five- and six-membered heterocyclic substituents at the 7-position. J Med Chem, 1990;33(4):1246–52, ISSN-0022-2623.

[11] Cooper CS, Klock PL, Chu DTW, Hardy DJ, Swanson RN, Plattner JJ Preparation and in vitro and in vivo evaluation of quinolones with selective activity against Gram-positive organisms. J Med Chem 1992;35(8):1392–8, ISSN-0022-2623.

[12] Culbertson TP, Domagala JM, Peterson P, Bongers S, Nichols JB. New 7-substituted quinolone antibacterial agents. The synthesis of 1-ethyl-1,4-dihydro-4-oxo-7-(2-thiazolyl and 4-thiazolyl)-3-quinolinecarboxylic acids. J Heterocyclic Chem 1987;24(6): 1509–20, ISSN-0022-152X.

[13] Culbertson TP, Sanchez JP, Gambino L, Sesnie JA. Quinolone antibacterial agents substituted at the 7-position with spiroamines. Synthesis and structure-activity relationships. J Med Chem 1990;33(8)2270–5, ISSN-0022-2623.

[14] Di Cesare P, Bousard D, Essiz M, Jacquet JP, Ledoussal B, Kiechel JR, Remuzon P, Kessler RE, Fung-Tomc J, Desiderio J. Fluoronaphthyridines and -quinolones as antibacterial agents. 5. Synthesis and antimicrobial activity of chiral 1-tert-butyl-6-fluoro-7-substituted-naphthyridones. J Med Chem 1992;35(22): 4205–13, ISSN-0022-2623.

[15] Domagala JM, Heifetz CL, Mich TF, Nichols JB. 1-Ethyl-7-[3-[(ethylamino)methyl]-1-pyrrolidinyl]-6,8-difluoro-1,4-dihydro-4-oxo-3-quinolinecarboxylic acid. New quinolone antibacterial with potent gram-positive activity. J Med Chem 1986;29(4): 445–8, ISSN-0022-2623.

[16] Domagala JM, Hagen SE, Heifetz CL, Hutt MO, Mich TF, Sanchez JP, Trehan AK. 7-Substituted 5-amino-1-cyclopropyl-6,8-difluoro-1,4-dihydro-4-oxo-3-quinolinecarboxylic acids: synthesis and biological activity of a new class of quinolone antibacterials. J Med Chem 1988;31(3):503–6, ISSN-0022-2623.

[17] Domagala JM, Bridges AJ, Culbertson TP, Gambino L, Hagen SE, Karrick G, Porter K, Sanchez JP, Sesnie J.A. Synthesis and biological activity of 5-amino- and 5-hydroxyquinolones, and the overwhelming influence of the remote N1-substituent in determining the structure-activity relationship. J Med Chem 1991;34(3):1142–54, ISSN-0022-2623.

[18] Domagala JM, Hagen SE, Joannides T, Kiely JS, Laborde E, Schroeder MC, Sesnie JA, Shapiro MA, Suto MJ, Vanderroest S. Quinolone antibacterials containing the new 7-[3-(1-aminoethyl)-1-pyrrolidinyl] side chain: the effects of the 1-aminoethyl moiety and its stereochemical configurations on potency and in vivo efficacy. J Med Chem 1993;36(7):871–82, ISSN-0022-2623.

[19] Frigola J, Peres J, Corbera J, Vano D, Merce R, Antoni T, Mas J, Valenti E. 7-Azetidinylquinolones as antibacterial agents. Synthesis and structure-activity relationships. J Med Chem 1993;36(7):801–10, ISSN-0022-2623.

[20] Frigola J, Torrens A, Castrillo JM, Vano D, Berrocal JM, Calvet C, Salgado L, Redondo J. 7-Azetidinylquinolones as antibacterial agents. 2. Synthesis and biological activity of 7-(2,3-disubstituted-1-azetidinyl)-4-oxoquinoline- and -1,8-naphthyridine-3-carboxylic acids. Properties and structure-activity relationships of quinolones with an azetidine moiety. J Med Chem 1994;37(24):4195–210, ISSN-0022-2623.

[21] Frigola J, Vano D, Torrens A, Gomez-Gomar A, Ortega E, Garcia-Granda S. 7-Azetidinylquinolones as antibacterial agents. 3. Synthesis, properties and structure-

activity relationships of the stereoisomers containing a 7-(3-amino-2-methyl-1-azetidinyl) moiety. J Med Chem 1995;38(7):1203–15, ISSN-0022-2623.

[22] Fukui H, Shibata T, Naito T, Nakano J, Maejima T, Senda H, Iwatani W, Tatsumi Y, Suda M, Arika T. Synthesis and antibacterial activity of novel 7-(3-substituted-3 or 4-trifluoromethyl-1-pyrrolidinyl)-8-methoxyfluoroquinolones. Bioorg Med Chem Lett 1988;8(20):2833–8, ISSN: 0960-894X.

[23] Hagen SE, Domagala JM, Heifetz CL, Sanchez JP, Solomon M. New quinolone antibacterial agents. Synthesis and biological activity of 7-(3,3- or 3,4-disubstituted-1-pyrrolidinyl)quinoline-3-carboxylic acids. J Med Chem 1990a;33(2):849–54, ISSN-0022-2623.

[24] Hagen ES, Domagala MJ. Synthesis of 5-methyl-4-oxo-quinolinecarboxylic acids. J Heterocyclic Chem 1990b;27(6):1609–16, ISSN-0022-152X.

[25] Hagen ES, Domagala JM, Heifetz CL, Johnson J. Synthesis and biological activity of 5-alkyl-1,7,8-trisubstituted-6-fluoroquinoline-3-carboxylic acids. J Med Chem 1991;3(3): 1155–61, ISSN-0022-2623.

[26] Hagen SE, Domagala JM, Gracheck SJ, Sesnie JA, Stier MA, Suto MJ. Synthesis and antibacterial activity of new quinolones containing a 7-[3-(1-amino-1-methylethyl)-1-pyrrolidinyl] moiety. Gram-positive agents with excellent oral activity and low side-effect potential. J Med Chem 1994;37(6):733–8, ISSN-0022-2623.

[27] Isao H, Attashi S.. Eur. Pat. Appl. EP 01 911 85, 1990.

[28] Itoh Y, Kato H. Ger. Offen DE 34 33 924 A1, 1984.

[29] Jose A, Fromtling RA, Bland JA, Pelak BA, Gilfillan EC. (Acyloxy)alkyl carbamate prodrugs of norfloxacin. J Med Chem 1991;34(1):78–81, ISSN-0022-2623.

[30] Kaziko A, Tsuyoshi K, Uemori S, Moriguchi A, Ikeda Y, Hirayama F, Yokoyama Y, Iwao E, Yakushiji T. Quinolone antimicrobial agents substituted with morpholines at the 7-position. Syntheses and structure-activity relationships. J Med Chem 1993;36(10): 1356–63, ISSN-0022-2623.

[31] Kondo H, Sakamato F, Kawakami K, Tsukamoto G. Studies on prodrugs. 7. Synthesis and antimicrobial activity of 3-formylquinolone derivatives. J Med Chem 1988;31(1): 3344–52, ISSN-0022-2623.

[32] Koga H, Itoh A, Murayama S. Structure-activity relationships of antibacterial 6,7- and 7,8-disubstituted 1-alkyl-1,4-dihydro-4-oxoquinoline-3-carboxylic acids. J Med Chem 1980;23(12):1358–1363, ISSN-0022-2623.

[33] Laborde E, Kiely JS, Culbertson TP, Lesheski LE. Quinolone antibacterials: synthesis and biological activity of carbon isosteres of the 1-piperazinyl and 3-amino-1-pyrrolidinyl side chains. J Med Chem 1993;36(14):1964–70, ISSN-0022-2623.

[34] Liu J, Guo H. Synthesis and antibacterial activity of 1-(substituted pyrrolyl)-7-(substituted amino)-6-fluoro-1,4-dihydro-4-oxo-3-quinolinecarboxylic acids. J Med Chem 1992;35(19):3469–73, ISSN-0022-2623.

[35] Moran BD, Ziegler BC, Dunne TS, KucK NA, Lin YI. Synthesis of novel 5-fluoro analogs of norfloxacin and ciprofloxacin. J Med Chem 1989;32(12):1313–8, ISSN-0022-2623.

[36] Myamoto T, Matsumoto J, Chiba K, Egawa H, Shibamori K, Minamida A, Nishimura Y, Okada H, Kataoka M. Pyridonecarboxylic acids as antibacterial agents. Part 14. Synthesis and structure-activity relationships of 5-substituted 6,8-difluoroquinolones, including sparfloxacin, a new quinolone antibacterial agent with improved potency. J Med Chem 1990;33(6):1645–56, ISSN-0022-2623.

[37] Ohta M, Koga H. Three-dimensional structure-activity relationships and receptor mapping of N1-substituents of quinolone antibacterials. J Med Chem 1991;34(1):131–9, ISSN-0022-2623.

[38] Pesson M. Ger. Offen Patent DE 28 409 10, 1979.

[39] Petersen U, Grohe K. Ger. Offen Patent DE 32 485 06, 1984b.

[40] Pintilie L, Oniscu C, Voiculescu Gh, Draghici C, Caproiu MT, Alexandru N, Paraschiv I, Damian E, Dobrovolschi D, Diaconu L. Synthesis and antibacterial activity of some novel fluoroquinolones. Romanian Biotechnol Lett 2003b;8(2):1197–204. ISSN 1224-5984.

[41] Pintilie L, Negut C, Oniscu C, Caproiu MT, Nechifor M, Iancu L, Ghiciuc C, Ursu R. Synthesis and antibacterial activity of some novel quinolones. Romanian Biotechnol Lett 2009b;14(5):4756–67, ISSN 1224-5984.

[42] Pintilie L, Nita S. RO *Patent application* RO A/01346, 07.12.2011a.

[43] Pintilie L, Nita S. RO *Patent application* RO A/01345, 07.12.2011b.

[44] Pintilie L, Dorobat O, Caproiu MT, Maganu M. Quinolone derivatives with activity against multi-drug resistant gram-positive microorganisms. Revista de chimie 20141;65(10):1176–81, ISSN 0034-7752.

[45] Pintilie L, Nicu AI, Stefaniu A, Deaconu M, Caproiu MT. RO *Patent application ROA*/ 00803/28.10.2014b.

[46] Radl S, Zikan V. Synthesis of some 1-aryl-1,4-dihydro-4-oxo-quinoline-3-carboxylic acids and their antibacterial activity. Collect. Czech Chem Commun 1989;54(8):2181–9, ISSN – 0010-0765.

[47] Remuzon P, Bouzard D, Di Cesare P, Essiz M, Jacquet JP, Kiechel JR, Ledoussal B, Kessler RE, Fung-Tomc J. Fluoronaphthyridines and -quinolones as antibacterial agents. 3. Synthesis and structure-activity relationships of new 1-(1,1-dimethyl-2-fluoroethyl), 1-[1-methyl-1-(fluoromethyl)-2-fluoroethyl], and 1-[1,1-(difluoromethyl)-2-fluoroethyl] substituted derivatives. J Med Chem 1991;34(1):29–37, ISSN-0022-2623.

[48] Renau TE, Sanchez JP, Gage JW, Dever JA, Shapiro MA, Gracheck SJ, Domagala JM. Structure–activity relationships of the quinolone antibacterials against mycobacteria: effect of structural changes at N-1 and C-7 J Med Chem 1996;39(3):799–835, ISSN-0022-2623.

[49] Reuman M, Daum SJ, Singh B, Wentland MP, Perni RB, Pennock P, Carabateas PM, Gruett MD, Saindane MT, Dorff PH, Coughlin SA, Sedlock DM, Rake JB, Lesher GY. Synthesis and antibacterial activity of some novel 1-substituted 1,4-dihydro-4-oxo-7-pyridinyl-3-quinolinecarboxylic acids. Potent antistaphylococcal agents. J Med Chem 1995;38(14):2531–40, ISSN-0022-2623.

[50] Rosen T, Chu DTW, Lico IM, Fernandes PB, Marsh K, Shen L, Cepa VG, Pernet AG. Design, synthesis, and properties of (4S)-7-(4-amino-2-substituted-pyrrolidin-1-yl)quinolone-3-carboxylic acids. J Med Chem 1988b;31(8):1598–611, ISSN-0022-2623.

[51] Sakamato F, Ikeda S, Kondo H, Tsukamoto G.. Studies on prodrugs. IV. Preparation and characterization of N-(5-substituted 2-oxo-1,3-dioxol-4-yl)methyl norfloxacin. Chem Pharm Bull1986;33(11):4870–7, ISSN- ISSN: 0009-2363.

[52] Sanchez JP, Bridges AJ, Bucsh R, Domagala JM, Gogliotti RD, Hagen SE, Heifetz CL, Joannides ET, Sesnie JC. New 8-(trifluoromethyl)-substituted quinolones. The benefits of the 8-fluoro group with reduced phototoxic risk. J Med Chem 1992a;35(2):361–7, ISSN-0022-2623.

[53] Sanchez JP, Domagala JM, Heifetz CL, Priebe SR, Sesnie JA, Trehan AK. Quinolone antibacterial agents. Synthesis and structure-activity relationships of a series of amino acid prodrugs of racemic and chiral 7-(3-amino-1-pyrrolidinyl)quinolones. Highly soluble quinolone prodrugs with in vivo pseudomonas activity. J Med Chem 1992b; 35(10):1764–73, ISSN-0022-2623.

[54] Sanchez JP. J Med Chem 1988;31(10):983–91, ISSN-0022-2623.

[55] Sanchez JP. J Med Chem 1995;38(10)4478–87, ISSN-0022-2623.

[56] Scriewer M, Petersen U, Grohe K. Eur. Pat. Appl EP 03 320 33, 1988a.

[57] Scriewer M, Petersen U, Grohe K. Ger. Offen Patent DE 3808 118, 1988b.

[58] Scott LD Quinolone antibacterial. In: Antibacterial Chemotherapeutic Agents, 1997, pp. 298-345, Blackie Academic & Professional, London, ISBN 10 0751402893.

[59] Segawa J, Kitano M, Kazuno K, Matsuoka M, Shirahase I, Ozaki M, Matsuda M, Tomii Y, Kise M. Studies on pyridonecarboxylic acids. 1. Synthesis and antibacterial evaluation of 7-substituted-6-halo-4-oxo-4H-[1,3]thiazeto[3,2-a]quinoline-3-carboxylic acids. J Med Chem 1992;35(25)4727–38, ISSN-0022-2623.

[60] Shongo A, Imamura M, Kimura Y, Yoshida A, Hayakawa I. Fluorocyclopropyl quinolones. 1. Synthesis and structure-activity relationships of 1-(2-fluorocyclopropyl)-3-pyridonecarboxylic acid antibacterial agents. J Med Chem 1993;36(22)3444–8, ISSN-0022-2623.

[61] Suto MJ, Domagala JM, Roland GE, Mailloux GB, Cohen MA. Fluoroquinolones: relationships between structural variations, mammalian cell cytotoxicity and antimicrobial activity. J Med Chem 1992;35(25):4745–50, ISSN-0022-2623.

[62] Taguchi M, Kondo H, Inoue Y, Kawahata Y, Jinbo Y, Sakamoto F, Tsukamoto G. Synthesis and antibacterial activity of new tetracyclic quinolone antibacterials. J Med Chem 1992;35(1):94–9, ISSN-0022-2623.

[63] Toshio U, Takamatsu M, Inoue Y, Kawahata Y, Iuchi K, Tsukamoto G. Synthesis of antimicrobial agents. 1. Syntheses and antibacterial activities of 7-(azole substituted)quinolones. J Med Chem 1987;30(120)2163–9, ISSN-0022-2623.

[64] Youichi Kimura Y, Atarashi S, Kawakami K, Sato K, Hayakawa I. Fluorocyclopropyl)quinolones. 2. Synthesis and stereochemical structure-activity relationships of chiral 7-(7-amino-5-azaspiro[2.4]heptan-5-yl)-1-(2-fluoro cyclopropyl) quinolone antibacterial agents. J Med Chem 1994;37(20)3344–52, ISSN-0022-2623.

[65] Wentland MP, Bailey DM, Cornett JB, Dobson RA, Powless RG, Wagner RB. Novel amino-substituted 3-quinolinecarboxylic acid antibacterial agents: synthesis and structure-activity relationships. J Med Chem 1984;27(9)1103–1, ISSN-0022-2623.

[66] Wentland MP, Lesher GY, Reuman M, Gruett MD, Singh B, Aldous SC, Dorff PH, Rake JB, Coughlin SA. Mammalian topoisomerase II inhibitory activity of 1-cyclopropyl-6,8-difluoro-1,4-dihydro-7-(2,6-dimethyl-4-pyridinyl)-4-oxo-3-quinolinecarboxylic acid and related derivatives. J Med Chem 1993;36(19):2801–9, ISSN-0022-2623.

[67] Ziegler Jr CB, Bitha P, Kuck NA, Fenton TJ, Petersen PJ, Lin YI. Synthesis and structure-activity relationships of new 7-[3-(fluoromethyl) piperazinyl]- and -(fluorohomopiperazinyl)quinolone antibacterials. J Med Chem 1990;33(1):142–6, ISSN-0022-2623.

[68] Ziegler Jr GB, Nydia AK, Strohmeyer TW, Lin YL. Synthesis and In vitro biological activity of some 7-(5-aminomethyl-2-isoxazolidinyl)quinolone-3-carboxylic acids. J Heterocyclic Chem 1990;27(6):2077–9, ISSN-0022-152X.

Chapter 4

Chitosan as a Biomaterial — Structure, Properties, and Electrospun Nanofibers

H. M. Ibrahim and E.M.R. El- Zairy

Additional information is available at the end of the chapter

http://dx.doi.org/10.5772/61300

Abstract

Chitosan is a polysaccharide derived from chitin; chitin is the second most abundant polysaccharide in the world, after cellulose. Chitosan is biocompatible, biodegradable and non-toxic, so that it can be usedin medicalapplications such as antimicrobial and wound healing biomaterials. It also used as chelating agent due to its ability to bind with cholesterol, fats, proteins and metal ions.

Chitosan is difficult to electrospun into a fibrous structure because it has a polycationic character in an acidic aqueous solution due to the many amino groups in its backbone. Fibrous structures were successfully formed by electrospinning chitosan solutions in 90 wt. % aqueous acetic acid solution or trifluoroacetic acid (TFA) or TFA/dichloromethane (DCM) in the presence of poly vinyl alcohol (PVA) or Poly ethylene oxide(PEO).Chitosan nanofibers are biocompatible and biodegradable, so they can used as hemostatic and wound healing materials.

Keywords: Chitosan, Biocompatibility, Biodegradability, Antimicrobial activity, Functionality, Nanofibers, Elecrtrospinning

1. Introduction

Chitosan is a polysaccharide derived from chitin; chitin is the second most abundant polysaccharide in the world, after cellulose. The presence of amino groups in the chitosan structure might be protonated-providing solubility in diluted acidic aqueous solutions, several remarkable properties of chitosan offered unique opportunities to the development of biomedical applications. The elucidation of their mechanism will lead to a better understanding of chitosan medical and pharmaceutical interest. The haemostatic activity of chitosan can also be related to the presence of positive charges on chitosan backbone. Due to its positive charges, chitosan can also interact with the negative part of cells membrane, which can lead to reorganization and an opening of the tight junction proteins, explaining the permeation enhancing property of this polysaccharide.

The polycationic nature of chitosan also allows explaining chitosan analgesic effects. Now, to explain chitosan biodegradability, it is important to remember that chitosan is not only a polymer bearing amino groups, but also a polysaccharide, which consequently contains breakable glycosidic bonds. Chitosan is actually degraded in vivo by several proteases, and mainly lysozyme.

Chitosan is biocompatible, biodegradable and non-toxic, so that it can be used as medical applications as antimicrobial and wound healing biomaterials. It used as chelating agent due to its ability to bind with cholesterol, fats, proteins and metal ions [1]

Due to chitosan's many attractive properties such as biodegradability, natural origin, abundance, reactivity, etc., it has many areas of application including medical, agricultural, food processing, nutritional enhancement, cosmetics, and waste and water treatment.

Chitosan is difficult to electrospun into a fibrous structure because it has a polycationic character in an acidic aqueous solution due to the many amino groups in its backbone. Fibrous structures were successfully formed by electrospinning chitosan solutions in 90 wt. % aqueous acetic acid solution or by using trifluoroacetic acid (TFA) or TFA/dichloromethane (DCM).

Since the electrospinning of chitosan itself proved to be difficult, chitosan was mixed with other synthetic or natural polymers, such as PEO or PVA.

Chitin and chitosan nanofibers with (50-500nm diameter) are biocompatible and biodegradable, so they can used as hemostatic and wound healing materials [2].

2. Chitosan

Chitosan is a polysaccharide derived from chitin. Its molecular weight is typically between 300-1000 kDa depending on the source of chitin. After cellulose, chitin is the second abounant natural polymer in the world. It is found in crustacean such as shrimps and crab [1, 3]

The main Sources of Chitin and Chitosan are : Insects (e.g. Cuticle, Ovipositors and Beetle cocoon), Crustaceans e.g. (Crab shell and Shrimp shell), Squid e.g. (*Ommastrephes* pen and Loligo stomach wall), Centric Diatoms e.g. (*Thalassiosira fluviatilis and* Algae) and Fungi e.g. (*Mucor rouxi* and *Aspergillis nidulans).*

Chemical structure of chitin made up of 1-4 linked 2-acetamido-2-deoxy-β-D-glucopyranose (Figure 1).

Although chitin is found naturally in large amounts through many sources, chitosan is only found in nature in limited quantities, such as in some fungi. The chitosan used in industrial or research applications is typically derived from chitin through the use of chemical or enzymatic treatments [4].

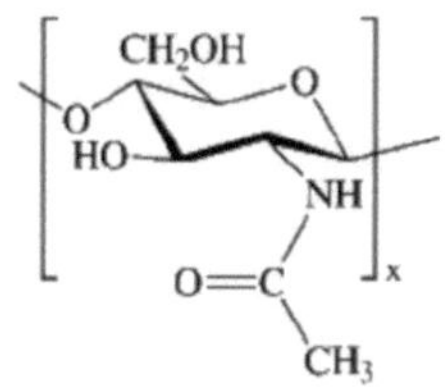

Figure 1. Chemical structure of chitin [4].

Chitosan is a copolymer of N-acetyl-D-glucose amine and D-glucose amine as shown in figure 2.It is a linear and semicrystals polymer [5, 6] chitosan has de acetylation degree at least 60% of glucose amine residue.(which corresponds to a deacetylation degree of 60). The deacetylation of chitin is conducted by chemical hydrolysis under severe alkaline conditions or by enzymatic hydrolysis in the presence of particular enzymes, among of chitin deacetylase [7, 8].

After cellulose, chitin is the second most abundant biopolymer [6] and is commonly found in invertebrates as crustacean shells or insect cuticles but also in some mushrooms envelopes, green algae cell walls, and yeasts [9-11]. At industrial scale, the two main sources of chitosan are crustaceans and fungal mycelia; the animal source shows however some drawbacks as seasonal, of limited supplies and with product variability which can lead to inconsistent physicochemical characteristics [12]. The mushroom source offers the advantage of a controlled production environment all year round that insures a better reproducibility of the resulting chitosan [13], chitosan is safe for both healthcare and biomedical application [5, 14]. The mushroom-extracted chitosan typically presents a narrower molecular mass distribution than the chitosan produced from seafood [14], and may also differ in terms of molecular mass, DD and distribution of deacetylated groups [13, 15]. Chitosan DD greatly varies between 60 and 100% while its molecular weight typically ranges from 300 to 1000 kDA [16], depending on the source and preparation. Chitosan oligomers can be prepared by degradation of chitosan using specific enzyme [5] or reagent as hydrogen peroxide [17].

After production, many different tools such as pH-potentiometric titration, IR-spectroscopy, viscosimetry, 1H NMR spectroscopy, UV-spectroscopy, and enzymatic degradation can determine chitosan properties [5, 6, 18].

2.1. The relationship between structure and properties

Chitosan differ from chitin by the presence of amino groups which appears in its solubility in dilute acids ($pH < 6$), and forming complexes with metal ions so that it can be used for waste water treatment and purification. [5, 6]. In contrast, practical applications of chitin are extremely limited due to its poor solubility, if any [19]. Interestingly, the aqueous solubility of chitosan is pH dependent allowing processability under mild conditions [20].

Chitosan with protonated amino groups becomes a polycation that can subsequently form ionic complexes with a wide variety of natural or synthetic anionic species [20], such as lipids, proteins, DNA and some negatively charged synthetic polymers as poly (acrylic acid) [19-22]. As a matter of fact, chitosan is the only positively charged, naturally occurring polysaccharide [19].

Chitosan molecules have both amino and hydroxyl groups so that it can form stable covalent bonds via several reactions such as etherification, esterification and reductive amination reactions [5, 6].

Chitosan have remarkable antibacterial activity [5, 23, 24], along with antifungal [11], mucoadhesive [25], analgesic [11] and haemostatic properties [26]. It can be biodegraded into non-toxic residues [27, 28] the rate of its degradation being highly related to the molecular mass of the polymer and its deacetylation degree – and has proved to some extent biocompatibility with physiological medium [29, 30]. All these singular features make chitosan an outstanding candidate for biomedical applications.

Chitosan, deacetylated form of chitin to at least 50% of the free amine form, has a heterogeneous chemical structure made up of both 1-4 linked 2-acetamido-2-deoxy-β-D-glucopyranose as well as 2-amino-2-deoxy-β-D-glucopyranose (Figure 2).

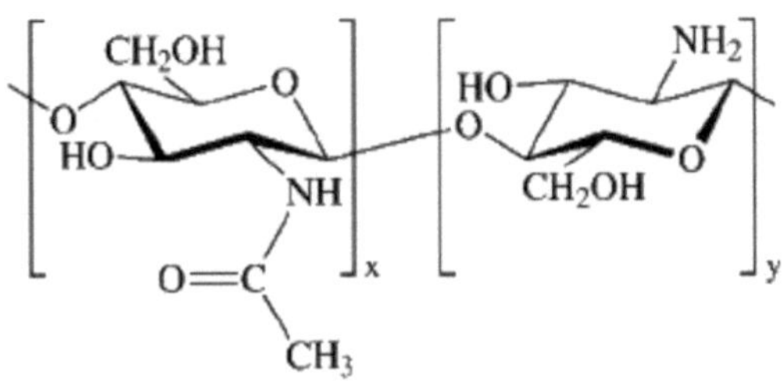

Figure 2. Chemical structure chitosan [4].

2.2. Chitin and chitosan production

Chitosan produced from crustacean shell such as crab and shrimp. These shells contains 30-40% proteins, 30-50% calcium carbonate and 20-30% chitin (etd.lsu.edu).

Production of chitosan involves four steps: demineralization, (DM), deproteinization (DP), decolorization (DC), and deacetylation (DA), as shown in Figure 3 (**etd.lsu.edu**).

The process for the deacetylation of chitin, obtained from crab or shrimp shells, to form chitosan is described in Figure 5 and generally produces a chitosan with 70% to 95% deacetylation [4].

3. Chitosan as biomaterial

Chitosan have several properties to be used in biomedical applications. It has positive charges in acidic medium, due to protonation of amino groups, and it can bind with negative residues in the mucin, that lead to improve mucoadhesive properties [5, 15].

http://dx.doi.org/10.5772/61300

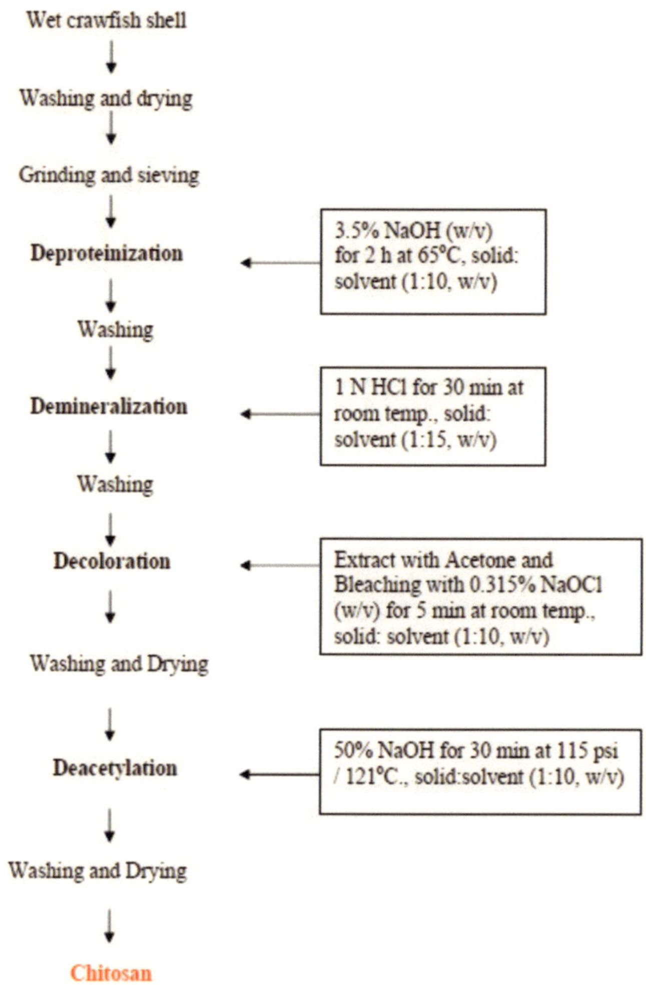

Figure 3. Chitosan production flow scheme [4, 31].

Also positive charges on chitosan can bind to negative charges on red blood cells (RBC) so that chitosan used as haemostatic agent [5, 32, 33].

Chitosan has two mechanisms to explain its antimicrobial activity. The first mechanism proposed that positive charges on chitosan could bind with negative charges at the bacterial cell surface, which alter permeability and leaks solutes outside the cells. The second one proposed that it could bind with bacterial DNA cell, which inhibit RNA synthesis [5].

The polycationic nature of chitosan also allows explaining chitosan analgesic effects. Indeed, the amino groups of the D-glucosamine residues can protonate in the presence of proton ions that are released in the inflammatory area, resulting in an analgesic effect [34].

Now, to explain chitosan biodegradability, it is important to remember that chitosan is not only a polymer bearing amino groups, but also a polysaccharide, which consequently contains breakable glycosidic bonds. Chitosan is actually degraded in vivo by several proteases, and mainly lysozyme [11, 35, 36]. Till now, eight human chitinases have been identified, three of them possessing enzymatic activity on chitosan [37]. The biodegradation of chitosan leads to the formation of non-toxic oligosaccharides of variable length. These oligosaccharides can be incorporated in metabolic pathways or be further excreted [38]. The degradation rate of chitosan is mainly related to its degree of deacetylation, but also to the distribution of N-acetyl D-glucosamine residues and the molecular mass of chitosan [39-41].

Chitosan shows biocompatibility in biomedical applications such as sutures and artificial skins [5, 6, 10, 34] and was notably approved by the Food and Drug Administration (FDA) for use in wound dressings [42]. However, the compatibility of chitosan with physiological medium depends on the preparation method (residual proteins could indeed cause allergic reactions) and on the DD – biocompatibility increases with DD increase. Chitosan actually proved to be more cytocompatible in vitro than chitin. Indeed, while the number of positive charges increases the interaction between cells and chitosan increases as well, which tends to improve biocompatibility [43].

Besides, some chemical modifications of chitosan structure could induce toxicity [35].

Production process of chitosan has great effect on chitosan properties because these processes control the degree of acetylation of chitosan, i.e. free amino groups that allow it to bind with negatively charged molecules [1, 4, 44].

Chitosan has several biological properties that make it an attractive material for use in medical applications. These properties include: biodegradability, lack of toxicity, anti-fungal effects, wound healing acceleration and immune system stimulation [4, 44-46].

4. Applications of chitosan and chitosan derivatives

Due to chitosan's many attractive properties such as biodegradability, natural origin, abundance, reactivity, etc., it has many areas of application including: medical, agricultural, food processing, nutritional enhancement, cosmetics, and waste and water treatment [4, 44].

4.1. Agricultural applications

The abundance, biodegradability, nontoxic, and natural origin of chitosan allow it to be safely used in agricultural applications because it can be used without concerns of pollution, disposal, or harm to consumers if ingested. Seed coating, leaf coating, fertilizer, and time released drug or fertilizer responses are some of the applications within agricultural where chitosan is utilized. The use of chitosan in these areas has shown to increase the amount of crops produced by improving germination, rooting, leaf growth, seed yield, and soil moisture retention, while reducing the occurrence of fungal infections and diseases [47].

4.2. Wastewater treatment applications

Chitosan's functional groups and natural chelating properties make chitosan useful in wastewater treatment by allowing for the binding and removal of metal ions such as copper, lead, mercury, and uranium from wastewater [4]. It can also be utilized to breakdown food particles that contain protein and remove dyes and other negatively charged solids from wastewater streams and processing outlets [47].

4.3. Food industry applications

Chitosan's chelating properties and high functionality make it valuable in several applications within the food industry such as binding with and removing certain elements, particles, and materials such as dyes and fats from foods. The antibacterial and antifungal properties found in chitosan can also be used during the storage and preservation of food [4, 46, 47].

4.4. Medical applications

Due to chitosan's ability to function in many forms it has many areas of interest within the medical industry including orthopedic and Periodontal Applications [44, 46]. Tissue engineering [44, 45, 47-49], Wound Healing [44, 45, 50, 51] and Drug Delivery [52, 53].

Some examples of biomedical applications of are artificial skin, surgical sutures, artificial blood vessels, controlled drug release, contact lens, eye humor fluid, bandages, sponges, burn dressings, blood cholesterol control, anti-inflammatory, tumor inhibition, anti-viral, dental plaque inhibition, bone healing treatment, wound healing accelerator, hemostatic agent, antibacterial agent, antifungal agent, weight loss effect [44].

5. Electrospinning of chitosan

Electrospinning is a process that utilizes a strong electrostatic field to obtain ultrafine fibers from a polymer solution accelerated towards the grounded collector due to the motion of charge carriers present in the solution in order to complete the electrical circuit. Electrospun fibers with their high surface area to volume ratio and small pores, are drawing interest in vast variety of applications, some being, filtration products, scaffolds for tissue engineering, wound dressings, drug release materials, fiber reinforcement composites, protective clothing [54-56].

5.1. History of electrospinning

In 1700s, influence of electrostatics was observed on water behavior and an electric charge influenced the excitation of dielectric liquid. This probably led to the invention of electrospinning to produce fibers in the early 1900s by Cooley and Morton. Cooley added rotatory electrode to the electrospinning jet. Formhals, in 1930, produce yarns by using electrospinning without spinneret [57] and patented his invention relating to the process and the apparatus. In 1940, Formhals patented another method for producing composite fiber webs from multiple polymer substrates by electrostatically spinning polymer fibers on a moving base substrate. In 1969, Taylor studied the shape of the polymer droplet produced at the tip of the needle when an electric field was applied and showed that it was a cone and the jets ejected from the vortices of the cone. This cone was later referred to as the 'Taylor cone'. The effects of electric field, experimental conditions and the factors affecting the atomization and fiber stability were studied [58]. For the fiber industries, one important consideration is the rate of fiber production. Electrospinning, compared to the popular industrial fiber spinning processes, has very low production rates [57]. Industrial dry spinning has a yarn take-up rate of 200– 1500 m min −1 while yarn fabricated from electrospinning has a take-up speed of 30 m min−1. Thus, before 1990, there was very little industrially oriented research interest found on electrospinning. Melt spinning being the preferred method for producing synthetic fibers, efforts were made to electrospin fibers using polymer melts, but difficulties were encountered in fabricating fibers with nanometer diameters and, therefore, little progress was made in this specific approach. Nevertheless, Dalton et al [59] recently succeeded in depositing electrospun polymer melt fibers directly on to cells to form layered tissue constructs for tissue engineering. This eliminated the introduction of cytotoxic solvents into the cell culture when the fibers were deposited. While there have been patents filed for various electrospinning set-ups since the 1900s, it is only in the last decade that academia got heavily involved in using electrospinning to fabricate various nano-fibrous assemblies for a range of potential applications.

Figure 4 shows a comparison of diameters between nanofibers, proteins, viruses and bacterial cells [60].

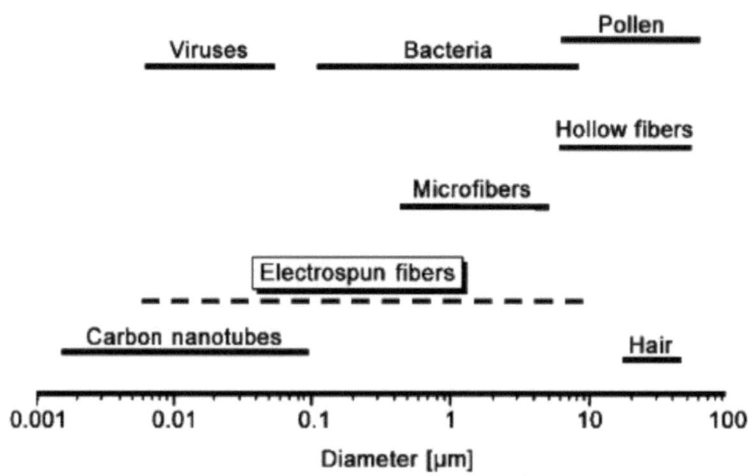

Figure 4. Comparison of the Diameters of Electrospun Fibers to those of Biological and Technological Objects [60].

5.2. Electrospinning process

Electrospinning as the production of fine fibers (either nano or micro) from polymer solutions by using high voltage electric field (kV) at room temperature and atmospheric conditions There are two electrospinning setups, vertical and horizontal [1, 61, 62].

Electrospinning devices, Figure 5, consists of three main componenet: high voltage electric field, spinneret and collecting electrode.[1, 63, 64].

Through electrospinning process, polymer solutions subjected to high voltage electric field that induce electric charge on its surface. At critical electric field, the repulsive electrical forces can overcome the surface tension and eject unstable charge jet from Taylor cone tip, which evaporate the solvent and leave the polymer [1, 65-68]. The jet is only stable at the tip of the spinneret and after that, instability starts. Thus, the electrospinning process offers a simplified technique for fiber formation.

Due to the critical voltage, applied potential reaches a critical value and the repulsive force within the charged solution exceeds surface tension and a jet erupts from the tip of the cone. These charged ions in the polymer jet move in response to the applied electric field towards the electrode of opposite polarity, thereby transferring tensile forces to the polymer jet making the latter undergo a chaotic motion or bending instability with whipping action. The jet moves towards the opposite charged collector, which collects the charged fibers. The jet ejected from the apex of the cone continues to thin down along the path of its travel towards the collector. As the jet travels through the atmosphere, the solvent evaporates, leaving behind a dry fiber on the collecting device. The structure formation happens on a millisecond scale[69]. An important step within production of the fibers is the elongation taking place within the jet with a strain rate as high as 10^4 sec^{-1}[55, 58, 70, 71].

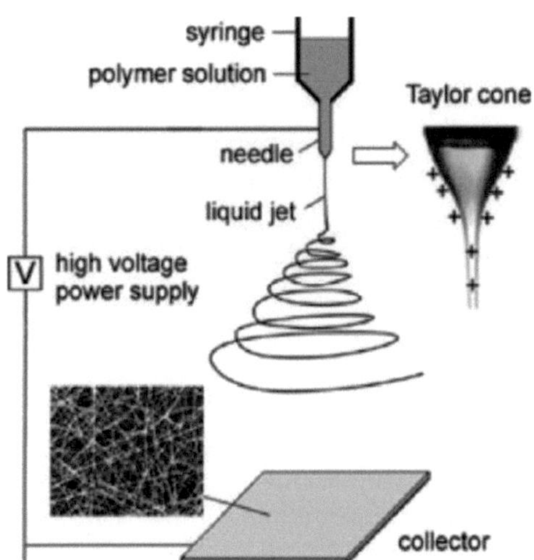

Figure 5. Schematic illustration of electrospinning setup [56].

A typical electrospinning setup only requires a high voltage power supply, a syringe, a flat tip needle and a conducting collector as shown in Figure 7. Electrospinning is able to produce continuous nanofibers from a wide range of materials. Nevertheless, there are many parameters, which affect the fiber morphology and properties in electrospinning. The main parameters are polymer parameters and processing conditions [54, 56, 72].

5.3. Effects of various parameters on electrospinning

There are several parameters affect the electrospinning process. These parameters are solution, process and ambient parameters [1, 56, 73]. In Table 1, there are summary of various parameters and their effects on fiber morphology[1].

Parameters	Effect on fiber morphology
Solution parameters	
Viscosity (η)	Low (η) generate beads, high (η) causes increase in fibre diameter and disappearance of beads
concentration	Fibre diameter increase with increasing of polymer concentration.
Molecular weight of polymer	The number of beads decrease, with increasing of molecular weight.
Conductivity	Decrease in fiber diameter with increase in conductivity.
Surface tension	Jets. Instability appears with high surface tension
Processing parameters	
Applied voltage	Decrease in fiber diameter with increase in voltage.
Distance between tip and collector	Generation of beads with too small and too large distance, minimum distance required for uniform fibers.
Feed rate/Flow rate	Decrease in fiber diameter with decrease in flow rate, generation of beads with too high flow rate.
Ambient parameters	
Humidity	High humidity results in circular pores on the fibers.
Temperature	Increase in temperature results in decrease in fiber diameter.

Table 1. Electrospinning Parameters (Solution, Processing and Ambient) and their Effects on Fiber Morphology [1].

5.4. Solvents used for electrospinning

Solvents play an important role in electrospinning to the dissolution of polymer in soluble solvent is the first step in the electrospinning process. These solvents should be volatile and have low boiling point such as chloroform, ethanol, dimethylformamide (DMF), trifluoroacetic acid (TEA), dichloromethane (DCM) [1, 74-76].

Solution properties such as viscosity and surface tension have great effect on the morphology of nanofibers [1, 77].

Basically, a solvent performs two crucial roles in electrospinning: Firstly, to dissolve the polymer molecules for forming the electrified jet. Secondly to carry the dissolved polymer molecules towards the collector [78], e.g. dimethylformamide, a dipolar aprotic solvent, has been successfully used as a solvent for electrospinning of poly (acrylonitrile) and its addition enhances the solution conductivity which is a prerequisite for the formation of bead free uniform fibers [79]. It was found that by increasing the concentration, there was a gradual decrease in surface tension of the solution, which favoured production of thinner fibers [80].

6. Electrospinning of chitosan solutions

Chitosan cannot form nanofibers through electrospinning process because its poly cationic nature due to the presence of many amino groups in its structure which increase solution surface tension [2, 81].

Fibrous structures were successfully formed by electrospinning chitosan solutions in 90wt% aqueous acetic acid solution [80] or by using trifluoroacetic acid (TFA) or TFA/dichloromethane (DCM) [78]. However, electrospinning conditions are relatively limited in terms of concentration, molecular weight, and degree of deacetylation [82]. The resultant chitosan fibers need to be cross-linked to maintain their structural integrity, as they can readily swell in aqueous solution [83].

Since the electrospinning of chitosan itself proved to be difficult. Chitosan was mixed with other synthetic or natural polymers, such as PEO in aqueous acid, PVA, aqueous acetic acid solution or aqueous acrylic acid solution, poly (lactic acid) (PLA) in trifluoroacetic acid/ methylene chloride mixture solvents or its copolymers in aqueous acetic acid solution, silk fibroin (SF) in formic acid, and collagen in 1,1,1,3,3,3,-hexafluoro-2-propanol/trifluoroacetic acid mixture solvent [2]. Several chitosan derivatives such as hexanoyl chitosan in Chloroform as a solvent, quaternized chitosan aqueous acetic acid solution or Water, N-carboxyethylchitosan in aqueous acrylic acid solution or water as solvent, and chitosan grafts with L-lactide or PEG oligomer in dimethylformamide/tetrahydrofuran solvent [2] were synthesized and electrospun with or without polymer additives, to improve the solubility and electrospinnability of chitosan

Chitin and chitosan nanofibers are biocompatible, biodegradable and nono-toxic so that it is used in biomedical applications such as antithrombogenic, hemostatic, and wound healing. The use of nanofibrous chitosan matrices is thus expected to mimic the natural ECM, in which cells attach, proliferate, and differentiate [2, 84, 85]. The use of nanofibrous chitosan matrices is thus expected to mimic the natural ECM, in which cells attach, proliferate, and differentiate.

An organic/inorganic composite scaffold of hydroxyapatite (HAp) and electrospun nanofibrous matrix was prepared by using chitosan/poly(vinyl alcohol) (CS/PVA) and N-carboxyethylchitosan/PVA (CECS/PVA) electrospun membranes, and HAp was formed in supersaturated $CaCl_2$ and KH_2PO_4 solution [86].

Xu et al was successful to prepare chitosan nanofibers used for enzyme immobilization by mixing its solution with polyvinyl alcohol (PVA) then added to sodium hydroxide solution for remaining the PVA and stabilizing chitosan nanofibers [87].

Chitosan nanofibers used for wound healing because it shows antibacterial activity against Staphylococcus aureus and Escherichia coli [87, 88]. In addition, chitosan nanofibers with (40-290 nm diameters) were prepared by electrospinning of its solution with polyethylene oxide (PEO) blended solution [89].

Quaternized chitosan (QCS) form nanofibers in the presence of polyvinyl alcohol (PVA) and poly vinyl pyrrolidone (PVP) as fiber aiding materials [90, 91].

Ultrafine fibers could be generated by controlling the addition of PEO in 2:1 or 1:1 mass ratios of CS to PEO from 4–6 wt% CS/PEO solutions to be used for cartilage tissue repair [92, 93].

Chitosan electrospun nanofibers are cellular biocompatible. Chitosan molecular and solvent used control the beads formation such as hexanoyl chitosan/poly lactide nanofibers in chloroform formed without beads. Also in chitosan/PVA nanofibers, beads formation decreased by increased the content of PVA repair [92, 94].

PVA are non-toxic, non-ionogenic and water-soluble polymer. Therefore, the nanofibrous materials prepared by electrospinning of CECS/PVA aqueous solutions, dissolved when put in contact with water. CECS / PVA mats stabilized by heating at 100°C. it is used in tissue schafolds applications [92, 94]. FTIR, XRD, and DSC studies demonstrated that there were strong intermolecular hydrogen bonds between the molecules of CS and PVA in the PVA/CS blend nanofibrous membranes [95]. SEM images showed that the morphology and diameter of the nanofibers were mainly affected by concentration of the blend solution (weight ratio of the blend) respectively [95]. It appears that electrospinning may emerge as a versatile method to manufacture CS fibers.

7. Nanofibers produced by electrospinning

7.1. Nanofiber morphology

Nanofibers produced by electrospinning have gained popularity in research in part due to their morphological characteristics. These nano-diameter fibers have high surface areas, small pore sizes and are able to be produced in three dimensional forms (Figure 6). Because the above mentioned characteristics can be modified through process parameters to suit individual applications and needs, electrospinning has become a growing topic among researchers [71].

7.2. Nanofiber properties

The properties associated with nanofibers can be traced back to both process parameters and morphological characteristics. For example electrospun fibers have small pores that are a result of the evaporation of the solvent used during the electrospinning process and these pores affect mechanical properties of the fibers such as tensile strength and Young's modulus [58]. Other

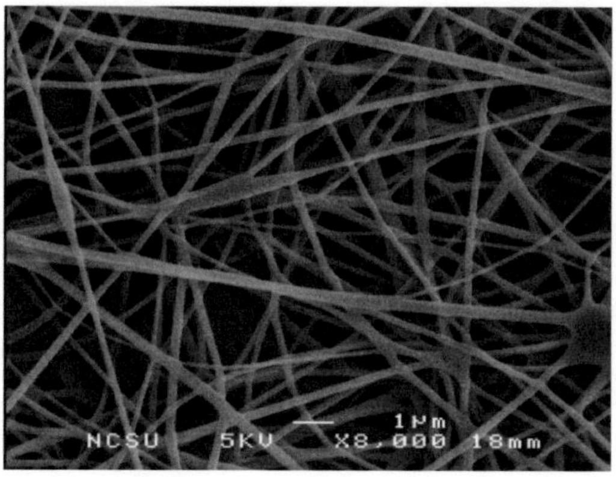

Figure 6. Scanning electron microscopy (SEM) image of electrospun poly (vinyl alcohol) produced on laboratory electrospinning setup.

studies have found that the physical properties of nanofibers tend to be somewhat inferior to that of their film and resin counterparts of a similar thickness. [65, 71] This is believed to be a result of lower crystallinity due to rapid evaporation of the solvent followed by rapid cooling, which occurs in the final stages of the electrospinning process [58].

7.3. Nanofiber applications

Characteristics such as large surface areas and the ability to be engineered in various forms have allowed nanofibers to be used in applications including: filtration [51], composite reinforcement [96], multifunctional membranes [51], tissue engineering scaffolds [3, 45, 51, 97, 98], wound dressings [50, 65, 99, 100], drug delivery [100-102], artificial organs [65, 103], and vascular grafts [65, 102-104]. Although all of these areas of interest are, still studied, biomedical applications for polymeric nanofibers have made up a majority of the new growth in the field of nanofiber research (Figure 7). [65] This growth is in part due to increased understanding of the human body, cellular structure, and the body's reaction to foreign materials.

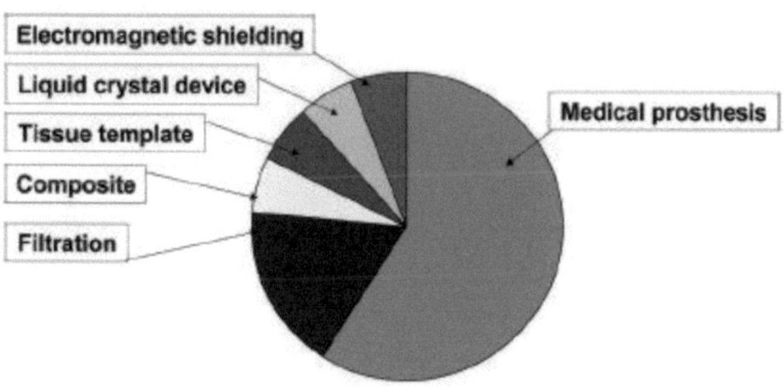

Figure 7. An estimation of the targeted nanofiber research fields based on the number of patent applications for electrospun nanofibers [65].

Researchers in the past have made attempts to electrospin chitosan in order to further utilize this material [33, 48, 49, 78, 80, 81, 84, 89, 93, 105]. Chitosan produces many challenges in being electrospun largely due to its high solution viscosity. Chitosan's rigid D-glucosamine structures, high crystallinity and ability to hydrogen bond lead to poor solubility in common organic solvents [105]. The smallest diameter fibers were reported using a poly(vinyl alcohol)/chitosan blend which resulted in nanofibers with average diameters between 20 and 100 nm [105]. Other studies have reported nearly defect free nanofibers, with slightly larger fiber diameters using a poly (ethylene oxide) (PEO)/chitosan blend [49, 89, 93, 105]. The successful electrospinning of pure chitosan has only been reported using a solvent system of 90 % acetic acid and a 7 wt. % concentration of chitosan [80].

The first successful reports of PEO/chitosan electrospun blends reported the electrospinning of nanofibers with diameters ranging from 40 to 290 nm, but that the most consistent and defect free fibers had an average diameter ranging from 200 to 250 nm (Spasova et al, 2004) Another study using a PEO/chitosan blend reported defect free nanofibers with diameters that ranged from 80 to 180 nm, but found that that the samples did not have consistent diameters. Using Fourier transform infrared spectroscopy and differential scanning calorimeter it was discovered that the two polymers had separated and the larger fibers largely consisted of PEO and the smaller fibers were predominately chitosan [93]. To further reduce the diameter of the electrospun PEO/chitosan blend fibers another research group introduced Triton X-100™ as a nonionic surfactant as well as dimethylsulphoxide as an additional solvent. These additions greatly improved the ability to electrospin PEO/chitosan blends with a high polymer concentration and produced fibers with diameters that ranged from 40 to 110 nm [49]. The same group also tested this nanomesh for cellular attachment and viability and found that cells more readily attached and were able to be sustained more efficiently than on a cast film of the same materials [49]. Another study was able to successfully electrospin PEO/chitosan blends with no additional additives, which resulted in fibers with an average diameter of 300 nm [48]. This group's main objective was to test the cellular viability of a chitosan blend in the electrospun nanomesh form. They concluded that chondrocyte cells showed good cell adhesion, proliferation and viability on the chitosan-based electrospun material. It also concluded that the electrospun material had a higher modulus compared to the control film made by solvent casting. [48]

Author details

H. M. Ibrahim[1*] and E.M.R. El- Zairy[2]

*Address all correspondence to: hmaibrahim@gmail.com

1 National Research Center, Textile Research Division, Dokki, Cairo, Egypt

2 Faculty of Applied Arts, Printing, Dyeing and Finishing Dept., Helwan Univ., Cairo, Egypt

References

[1] Bhardwaj, N. and S.C. Kundu, *Electrospinning: a fascinating fiber fabrication technique.* Biotechnology advances, 2010. 28(3): p. 325-347.

[2] Lee, K.Y., et al., *Electrospinning of polysaccharides for regenerative medicine.* Advanced Drug Delivery Reviews, 2009. 61(12): p. 1020-1032.

[3] Dvir, T., O. Tsur-Gang, and S. Cohen, *"Designer" scaffolds for tissue engineering and regeneration.* Israel journal of chemistry, 2005. 45(4): p. 487-494.

[4] Hudson, S.M. and D.W. Jenkins, *Chitin and chitosan, encyclopedia of polymer science and technology,* 2001, NJ: Wiley Interscience.

[5] Croisier, F. and C. Jérôme, *Chitosan-based biomaterials for tissue engineering.* European Polymer Journal, 2013. 49(4): p. 780-792.

[6] Rinaudo, M., *Chitin and chitosan: properties and applications.* Progress in polymer science, 2006. 31(7): p. 603-632.

[7] Jayakumar, R., et al., *Biomedical applications of chitin and chitosan based nanomaterials—A short review.* Carbohydrate Polymers, 2010. 82(2): p. 227-232.

[8] Venkatesan, J. and S.-K. Kim, *Chitosan composites for bone tissue engineering—An overview.* Marine drugs, 2010. 8(8): p. 2252-2266.

[9] Rane, K.D. and D.G. Hoover, *Production of chitosan by fungi.* Food biotechnology, 1993. 7(1): p. 11-33.

[10] Aranaz, I., R. Harris, and A. Heras, *Chitosan amphiphilic derivatives. Chemistry and applications.* Current Organic Chemistry, 2010. 14(3): p. 308.

[11] Aranaz, I., et al., *Functional characterization of chitin and chitosan.* Current Chemical Biology, 2009. 3(2): p. 203-230.

[12] Kannan, M., et al., *Production and characterization of mushroom chitosan under solid-state fermentation conditions.* Adv Biol Res, 2010. 4(1): p. 10-13.

[13] Wu, T., et al., *Chitin and chitosan value-added products from mushroom waste.* Journal of agricultural and food chemistry, 2004. 52(26): p. 7905-7910.

[14] Riva, R., et al., *Chitosan and chitosan derivatives in drug delivery and tissue engineering,* in *Chitosan for biomaterials II*2011, Springer. p. 19-44.

[15] Teng, W.L., et al., *Concurrent production of chitin from shrimp shells and fungi.* Carbohydrate research, 2001. 332(3): p. 305-316.

[16] Liu, X., et al., *Chitosan-based biomaterials for tissue repair and regeneration,* in *Chitosan for Biomaterials II*2011, Springer. p. 81-127.

[17] Yong, Z., *Study on the Preparation of Chitosan Oligomer through the Chitosan Degraded by Hydrogen Peroxide.* Journal of Anhui Agricultural Sciences, 2011. 21: p. 213.

[18] Balázs, N. and P. Sipos, *Limitations of pH-potentiometric titration for the determination of the degree of deacetylation of chitosan.* Carbohydrate research, 2007. 342(1): p. 124-130.

[19] Pavinatto, F.J., L. Caseli, and O.N. Oliveira Jr, *Chitosan in nanostructured thin films.* Biomacromolecules, 2010. 11(8): p. 1897-1908.

[20] Madihally, S.V. and H.W. Matthew, *Porous chitosan scaffolds for tissue engineering.* Biomaterials, 1999. 20(12): p. 1133-1142.

[21] Takahashi, T., et al., *Characteristics of polyion complexes of chitosan with sodium alginate and sodium polyacrylate.* International Journal of Pharmaceutics, 1990. 61(1): p. 35-41.

[22] Kim, T.-H., et al., *Chemical modification of chitosan as a gene carrier in vitro and in vivo.* Progress in polymer science, 2007. 32(7): p. 726-753.

[23] Sudarshan, N., D. Hoover, and D. Knorr, *Antibacterial action of chitosan.* Food biotechnology, 1992. 6(3): p. 257-272.

[24] Ong, S.-Y., et al., *Development of a chitosan-based wound dressing with improved hemostatic and antimicrobial properties.* Biomaterials, 2008. 29(32): p. 4323-4332.

[25] Lehr, C.-M., et al., *In vitro evaluation of mucoadhesive properties of chitosan and some other natural polymers.* International Journal of Pharmaceutics, 1992. 78(1): p. 43-48.

[26] Yang, J., et al., *Effect of chitosan molecular weight and deacetylation degree on hemostasis.* Journal of Biomedical Materials Research Part B: Applied Biomaterials, 2008. 84(1): p. 131-137.

[27] Bagheri-Khoulenjani, S., S. Taghizadeh, and H. Mirzadeh, *An investigation on the short-term biodegradability of chitosan with various molecular weights and degrees of deacetylation.* Carbohydrate Polymers, 2009. 78(4): p. 773-778.

[28] Vårum, K.M., et al., *In vitro degradation rates of partially N-acetylated chitosans in human serum.* Carbohydrate research, 1997. 299(1): p. 99-101.

[29] VandeVord, P.J., et al., *Evaluation of the biocompatibility of a chitosan scaffold in mice.* Journal of Biomedical Materials Research, 2002. 59(3): p. 585-590.

[30] Sashiwa, H. and S.-i. Aiba, *Chemically modified chitin and chitosan as biomaterials.* Progress in polymer science, 2004. 29(9): p. 887-908.

[31] No, H.K. and S.P. Meyers, *Preparation and characterization of chitin and chitosan—a review.* Journal of aquatic food product technology, 1995. 4(2): p. 27-52.

[32] Smith, J., E. Wood, and M. Dornish, *Effect of chitosan on epithelial cell tight junctions.* Pharmaceutical Research, 2004. 21(1): p. 43-49.

[33] Park, W.H., et al., *Effect of chitosan on morphology and conformation of electrospun silk fibroin nanofibers.* Polymer, 2004. 45(21): p. 7151-7157.

[34] Thanou, M., J. Verhoef, and H. Junginger, *Oral drug absorption enhancement by chitosan and its derivatives.* Advanced Drug Delivery Reviews, 2001. 52(2): p. 117-126.

[35] Dash, M., et al., *Chitosan—A versatile semi-synthetic polymer in biomedical applications.* Progress in polymer science, 2011. 36(8): p. 981-1014.

[36] Kean, T. and M. Thanou, *Chitin and chitosan—sources, production and medical applications.* Desk reference of natural polymers, their sources, chemistry and applications, Kentus Books, London, 2009: p. 327-361.

[37] Funkhouser, J.D. and N.N. Aronson, *Chitinase family GH18: evolutionary insights from the genomic history of a diverse protein family.* BMC evolutionary biology, 2007. 7(1): p. 96.

[38] Pangburn, S., P. Trescony, and J. Heller, *Lysozyme degradation of partially deacetylated chitin, its films and hydrogels.* Biomaterials, 1982. 3(2): p. 105-108.

[39] Aiba, S.-i., *Studies on chitosan: 4. Lysozymic hydrolysis of partially N-acetylated chitosans.* International journal of biological macromolecules, 1992. 14(4): p. 225-228.

[40] Tomihata, K. and Y. Ikada, *In vitro and in vivo degradation of films of chitin and its deacetylated derivatives.* Biomaterials, 1997. 18(7): p. 567-575.

[41] Zhang, H. and S.H. Neau, *In vitro degradation of chitosan by a commercial enzyme preparation: effect of molecular weight and degree of deacetylation.* Biomaterials, 2001. 22(12): p. 1653-1658.

[42] Wedmore, I., et al., *A special report on the chitosan-based hemostatic dressing: experience in current combat operations.* Journal of Trauma and Acute Care Surgery, 2006. 60(3): p. 655-658.

[43] Chatelet, C., O. Damour, and A. Domard, *Influence of the degree of acetylation on some biological properties of chitosan films.* Biomaterials, 2001. 22(3): p. 261-268.

[44] Şenel, S. and S.J. McClure, *Potential applications of chitosan in veterinary medicine.* Advanced Drug Delivery Reviews, 2004. 56(10): p. 1467-1480.

[45] Di Martino, A., M. Sittinger, and M.V. Risbud, *Chitosan: a versatile biopolymer for orthopaedic tissue-engineering.* Biomaterials, 2005. 26(30): p. 5983-5990.

[46] Khor, E. and L.Y. Lim, *Implantable applications of chitin and chitosan.* Biomaterials, 2003. 24(13): p. 2339-2349.

[47] Li, Q., et al., *Applications and properties of chitosan.* Journal of Bioactive and Compatible Polymers, 1992. 7(4): p. 370-397.

[48] Subramanian, A., et al., *Preparation and evaluation of the electrospun chitosan/PEO fibers for potential applications in cartilage tissue engineering.* Journal of Biomaterials Science, Polymer Edition, 2005. 16(7): p. 861-873.

[49] Bhattarai, N., et al., *Electrospun chitosan-based nanofibers and their cellular compatibility.* Biomaterials, 2005. 26(31): p. 6176-6184.

[50] Ueno, H., T. Mori, and T. Fujinaga, *Topical formulations and wound healing applications of chitosan.* Advanced Drug Delivery Reviews, 2001. 52(2): p. 105-115.

[51] Ma, Z., et al., *Potential of nanofiber matrix as tissue-engineering scaffolds.* Tissue engineering, 2005. 11(1-2): p. 101-109.

[52] Jayakumar, R., et al., *Graft copolymerized chitosan—present status and applications.* Carbohydrate Polymers, 2005. 62(2): p. 142-158.

[53] Prabaharan, M. and J. Mano, *Chitosan-based particles as controlled drug delivery systems.* Drug delivery, 2004. 12(1): p. 41-57.

[54] Fujihara, K., et al., *An introduction to electrospinning and nanofibers.* National University of Singapore, 2005.

[55] Reneker, D.H., et al., *Bending instability of electrically charged liquid jets of polymer solutions in electrospinning.* Journal of Applied physics, 2000. 87(9): p. 4531-4547.

[56] Li, D. and Y. Xia, *Electrospinning of nanofibers: reinventing the wheel?* Advanced materials, 2004. 16(14): p. 1151-1170.

[57] Teo, W. and S. Ramakrishna, *A review on electrospinning design and nanofibre assemblies.* Nanotechnology, 2006. 17(14): p. R89.

[58] Subbiah, T., et al., *Electrospinning of nanofibers.* Journal of Applied Polymer Science, 2005. 96(2): p. 557-569.

[59] Dalton, P.D., et al., *Direct in vitro electrospinning with polymer melts.* Biomacromolecules, 2006. 7(3): p. 686-690.

[60] Greiner, A. and J.H. Wendorff, *Electrospinning: a fascinating method for the preparation of ultrathin fibers.* Angewandte Chemie International Edition, 2007. 46(30): p. 5670-5703.

[61] Kidoaki, S., I.K. Kwon, and T. Matsuda, *Mesoscopic spatial designs of nano-and microfiber meshes for tissue-engineering matrix and scaffold based on newly devised multilayering and mixing electrospinning techniques.* Biomaterials, 2005. 26(1): p. 37-46.

[62] Stankus, J.J., et al., *Hybrid nanofibrous scaffolds from electrospinning of a synthetic biodegradable elastomer and urinary bladder matrix.* Journal of Biomaterials Science, Polymer Edition, 2008. 19(5): p. 635-652.

[63] Liang, D., B.S. Hsiao, and B. Chu, *Functional electrospun nanofibrous scaffolds for biomedical applications.* Advanced Drug Delivery Reviews, 2007. 59(14): p. 1392-1412.

[64] Sill, T.J. and H.A. von Recum, *Electrospinning: applications in drug delivery and tissue engineering*. Biomaterials, 2008. 29(13): p. 1989-2006.

[65] Huang, Z.-M., et al., *A review on polymer nanofibers by electrospinning and their applications in nanocomposites*. Composites science and technology, 2003. 63(15): p. 2223-2253.

[66] Taylor, G. *Disintegration of water drops in an electric field*. in *Proceedings of the Royal Society of London A: Mathematical, Physical and Engineering Sciences*. 1964. The Royal Society.

[67] Taylor, G. *Electrically driven jets*. in *Proceedings of the Royal Society of London A: Mathematical, Physical and Engineering Sciences*. 1969. The Royal Society.

[68] Adomavičiūtė, E. and R. Milašius, *The influence of applied voltage on poly (vinyl alcohol) (PVA) nanofibre diameter*. Fibres & Textiles in Eastern Europe, 2007(5-6 (64)): p. 69--72.

[69] Dersch, R., et al., *Electrospun nanofibers: Internal structure and intrinsic orientation*. Journal of Polymer Science Part A: Polymer Chemistry, 2003. 41(4): p. 545-553.

[70] Shin, Y., et al., *Electrospinning: A whipping fluid jet generates submicron polymer fibers*. Applied physics letters, 2001. 78(8): p. 1149-1151.

[71] Frenot, A. and I.S. Chronakis, *Polymer nanofibers assembled by electrospinning*. Current opinion in colloid & interface science, 2003. 8(1): p. 64-75.

[72] Lyons, J., C. Li, and F. Ko, *Melt-electrospinning part I: processing parameters and geometric properties*. Polymer, 2004. 45(22): p. 7597-7603.

[73] Chong, E., et al., *Evaluation of electrospun PCL/gelatin nanofibrous scaffold for wound healing and layered dermal reconstitution*. Acta biomaterialia, 2007. 3(3): p. 321-330.

[74] Son, W.K., et al., *Electrospinning of ultrafine cellulose acetate fibers: studies of a new solvent system and deacetylation of ultrafine cellulose acetate fibers*. Journal of Polymer Science Part B: Polymer Physics, 2004. 42(1): p. 5-11.

[75] Wannatong, L., A. Sirivat, and P. Supaphol, *Effects of solvents on electrospun polymeric fibers: preliminary study on polystyrene*. Polymer International, 2004. 53(11): p. 1851-1859.

[76] Veleirinho, B., M.F. Rei, and J. Lopes-DA-Silva, *Solvent and concentration effects on the properties of electrospun poly (ethylene terephthalate) nanofiber mats*. Journal of Polymer Science Part B: Polymer Physics, 2008. 46(5): p. 460-471.

[77] Yang, Q., et al., *Influence of solvents on the formation of ultrathin uniform poly (vinyl pyrrolidone) nanofibers with electrospinning*. Journal of Polymer Science Part B: Polymer Physics, 2004. 42(20): p. 3721-3726.

[78] Ohkawa, K., et al., *Electrospinning of chitosan*. Macromolecular Rapid Communications, 2004. 25(18): p. 1600-1605.

[79] Bhattarai, S.R., et al., *Novel biodegradable electrospun membrane: scaffold for tissue engineering.* Biomaterials, 2004. 25(13): p. 2595-2602.

[80] Geng, X., O.-H. Kwon, and J. Jang, *Electrospinning of chitosan dissolved in concentrated acetic acid solution.* Biomaterials, 2005. 26(27): p. 5427-5432.

[81] Min, B.-M., et al., *Chitin and chitosan nanofibers: electrospinning of chitin and deacetylation of chitin nanofibers.* Polymer, 2004. 45(21): p. 7137-7142.

[82] De Vrieze, S., et al., *Electrospinning of chitosan nanofibrous structures: feasibility study.* Journal of Materials Science, 2007. 42(19): p. 8029-8034.

[83] Schiffman, J.D. and C.L. Schauer, *One-step electrospinning of cross-linked chitosan fibers.* Biomacromolecules, 2007. 8(9): p. 2665-2667.

[84] Jiang, H., et al., *Preparation and characterization of ibuprofen-loaded poly (lactide-co-glycolide)/poly (ethylene glycol)-g-chitosan electrospun membranes.* Journal of Biomaterials Science, Polymer Edition, 2004. 15(3): p. 279-296.

[85] CHU, B. and W. CHEN, *Preparation and characterization of ibuprofen-loaded poly (lactide-co-glycolide)/poly (ethylene glycol)-g-chitosan electrospun membranes.*

[86] Yang, D., et al., *In Situ Mineralization of Hydroxyapatite on Electrospun Chitosan-Based Nanofibrous Scaffolds.* Macromolecular bioscience, 2008. 8(3): p. 239-246.

[87] Xu, S., et al., *Electrospinning of native cellulose from nonvolatile solvent system.* Polymer, 2008. 49(12): p. 2911-2917.

[88] Ignatova, M., et al., *Electrospun nano-fibre mats with antibacterial properties from quaternised chitosan and poly (vinyl alcohol).* Carbohydrate research, 2006. 341(12): p. 2098-2107.

[89] Spasova, M., et al., *Preparation of chitosan-containing nanofibres by electrospinning of chitosan/poly (ethylene oxide) blend solutions.* e-Polymers, 2004. 4(1): p. 624-635.

[90] Sun, K. and Z. Li, *Preparations, properties and applications of chitosan based nanofibers fabricated by electrospinning.* Express Polymer Letters, 2011. 5(4): p. 342-361.

[91] Pillai, C. and C.P. Sharma, *Electrospinning of chitin and chitosan nanofibres.* Trends in Biomaterials and Artificial Organs, 2009. 22(3): p. 179-201.

[92] Pillai, C., W. Paul, and C.P. Sharma, *Chitin and chitosan polymers: Chemistry, solubility and fiber formation.* Progress in polymer science, 2009. 34(7): p. 641-678.

[93] Duan, B., et al., *Electrospinning of chitosan solutions in acetic acid with poly (ethylene oxide).* Journal of Biomaterials Science, Polymer Edition, 2004. 15(6): p. 797-811.

[94] Mincheva, R., N. Manolova, and I. Rashkov, *Bicomponent aligned nanofibers of N-carboxyethylchitosan and poly (vinyl alcohol).* European Polymer Journal, 2007. 43(7): p. 2809-2818.

[95] Jia, Y.-T., et al., *Fabrication and characterization of poly (vinyl alcohol)/chitosan blend nanofibers produced by electrospinning method.* Carbohydrate Polymers, 2007. 67(3): p. 403-409.

[96] Kim, C.W., et al., *Preparation of submicron-scale, electrospun cellulose fibers via direct dissolution.* Journal of Polymer Science Part B: Polymer Physics, 2005. 43(13): p. 1673-1683.

[97] Schindler, M., et al., *A synthetic nanofibrillar matrix promotes in vivo-like organization and morphogenesis for cells in culture.* Biomaterials, 2005. 26(28): p. 5624-5631.

[98] Wang, Y.K., T. Yong, and S. Ramakrishna, *Nanofibres and their influence on cells for tissue regeneration.* Australian journal of chemistry, 2005. 58(10): p. 704-712.

[99] Rho, K.S., et al., *Electrospinning of collagen nanofibers: effects on the behavior of normal human keratinocytes and early-stage wound healing.* Biomaterials, 2006. 27(8): p. 1452-1461.

[100] Katti, D.S., et al., *Bioresorbable nanofiber-based systems for wound healing and drug delivery: Optimization of fabrication parameters.* Journal of Biomedical Materials Research Part B: Applied Biomaterials, 2004. 70(2): p. 286-296.

[101] Wu, X., L. Wang, and Y. Huang, *Application of electrospun ethyl cellulose fibers in drug release systems.* Acta Polymerica Sinica, 2006(2): p. 264-268.

[102] Miller, D.C., T.J. Webster, and K.M. Haberstroh, *Technological advances in nanoscale biomaterials: the future of synthetic vascular graft design.* Expert review of medical devices, 2004. 1(2): p. 259-268.

[103] Nerem, R., *Tissue engineering of vascular prosthetic grafts.* Nature Medicine, 1999. 5(10): p. 1118-1118.

[104] Stitzel, J., et al., *Controlled fabrication* of a biological vascular substitute. Biomaterials, 2006. 27(7): p. 1088-1094.

[105] Li, L. and Y.-L. Hsieh, Chitosan bicomponent nanofibers and nanoporous fibers. Carbohydrate research, 2006. 341(3): p. 374-381.

Chapter 5

Nisin

Angela Faustino Jozala,
Letícia Celia de Lencastre Novaes and
Adalberto Pessoa Junior

Additional information is available at the end of the chapter

http://dx.doi.org/10.5772/60932

Abstract

Antimicrobial peptides (AMPs) are small cationic peptides which protect their hosts against bacteria, protozoa, viruses, and fungi. Bacterial AMPs are called bacteriocins, and are produced by both Gram-positive and Gram-negative bacteria. Because of their high potency and specificity, bacteriocins are considered as promising antimicrobial agents for different applications, including food preservation and infection treatment; specially the ones produced by acid lactic bacteria species (Gram-positive). Nisin is the most intensively studied and used bacteriocin, it is found commercially available and its use is regulated in over 50 countries. Therefore, special attention is given to this bacteriocin.

Keywords: nisin, *Lactococcus lactis*, antimicrobial

1. Introduction

Antimicrobial peptides (AMPs) are small cationic peptides that protect their hosts against bacteria, protozoa, viruses, and fungi [1, 2]. Some of these peptides have also demonstrated a cytotoxic activity against tumor cells and sperm [3]. These peptides are produced by several forms of life, including bacteria, insects, plants, and vertebrates, and they have been recognized as ancient evolutionary molecules that have been effectively preserved in mammals [2, 4].

These evolutionarily conserved peptides in general constitute a highly heterogeneous group of molecules, which share common features, as the small size (20–50 aa) and cationic and amphiphilic or hydrophobic properties [4]. Since APMs have both a hydrophobic and hydrophilic side, they are soluble in aqueous environments yet also enter lipid-rich membranes [1].

AMPs demonstrate being effective against a broad range of microorganisms, including Gram-negative and Gram-positive bacteria, fungi, and viruses [1]. In higher organisms, AMPs contribute to innate immunity, serve as a first defense line against harmful microorganisms, and may be increased with inflammation and injury in humans [1, 4]. In bacteria, the production of AMPs provides a competitive advantage for the producer in certain ecological niches, being a successful strategy to decrease the numbers of competitors to obtain more nutrients [4, 5].

Bacterial AMPs are called bacteriocins and are produced by both Gram-positive and Gram-negative bacteria. However, there are some important differences between eukaryotic AMPs and bacteriocins. Bacteriocins are often very potent, acting at pico- to nanomolar concentrations, whereas micromolar concentrations are required for the activity of eukaryotic AMPs. Most bacteriocins have a very narrow target spectrum, that is, being active against only a few species/genera closely related to the producer, whereas eukaryotic AMPs are generally less specific with a broad target spectrum [4].

Bacteriocins are often confused in the literature with antibiotics. Antibiotics are secondary metabolites synthesized by enzymes and have clinical application. Bacteriocins are ribosomally synthesized and do not alter the flora of the intestinal tract since they are inactivated by digestive enzymes [5].

Table 1 shows the main differences between bacteriocins and antibiotics, based on the synthesis, mode of action, antimicrobial spectrum, toxicity, and resistance mechanism [6].

Characteristic	Bacteriocin	Antibiotic
Application	Food	Clinic
Synthesis	Ribosomal	Enzymes
Production	Primary metabolism	Secondary metabolism
Activity	Limited spectrum	Wide spectrum
Action	Cytoplasmic membrane	Several
Toxicity	Unknown	Yes
Microbial resistance	There are some strains	There are some strains

Table 1. Major characteristics that differentiate bacteriocins of antibiotics [6].

More than 99% of bacteria can produce at least one bacteriocin, most of which are not identified. These substances may be produced spontaneously or induced and the producers are immune to it [7]. Bacteriocins are classified according to the bacterial spectrum, molecular weight, chemical structure, and mode of action [8].

http://dx.doi.org/10.5772/60932

There are two important databases relative to bacterions. One is the BACTIBASE, an open-access data repository of bacteriocin, designed for the characterization of bacteriocins. BACTIBASE is developed by the Functional Proteomics and Alimentary Bio-preservation Unit at the Institute of Applied Biological Sciences Tunis (ISSBAT), Tunisia, in collaboration with Nutraceuticals and Functional Foods Institute (INAF), Laval University, Canada (http://bactibase.pfba-lab-tun.org/main.php) [9]. The BACTIBASE contains over 200 bacteriocins sequences, most of which are the products of Gram-positive bacteria, particularly lactic acid bacteria [10].

The other database is BAGEL, a web-based bacteriocin mining tool that helps to determine the presence of bacteriocins gene from a GenBank file based on a database containing information of known bacteriocins and adjacent genes involved in bacteriocin activity (http://bagel2.molgenrug.nl/) [9]. In Gram-negative bacteria, most bacteriocins have been characterized from *Escherichia coli* and other enterobacteria, and they are often referred to as microcins (small peptides, <10 kDa) or colicins (larger peptides, 25–80 kDa) [4]. The spectrum of activity manifested by bacteriocins of Gram-negative bacteria is narrower than those produced by Gram-positive bacteria [11]. Microcins show tolerance to heat and extreme pH and are divided into two subgroups [4, 5]:

a. Class I: low molecular weight (<5 kDa) and contain posttranslational modifications. Some members of this class are microcin B17, C7, and J25.

b. Class II: larger than class I (5–20 kDa) and has little or no posttranslational modifications. This subclass includes microcin E492, colicin V, and H47.

The colicins are synthesized by over half of *E. coli* strains and also by *Yersinia pestis* (pesticins), *Serratia marcescens* (marcescins), and bacteria of genus *Shigella*, *Klebsiella* (klebicins), and *Pseudomonas* (pyocins) [11].

The bacteriocins of Gram-positive bacteria are divided into four classes, according to their genetic and biochemical characteristics [6, 12, 13], being lactic acid bacteria frequently found as producers. The classes are presented as follows:

Class I (lantibiotics): constituted by thermostable low-molecular peptides (<5 kDa) with 19–38 amino acid residues, posttranslationally modified and which have highly specific amino acid in their composition, as lanthionine and β-methyl lanthionine. Class I can be divided into subclasses based on the structure and mode of action of the bacteriocin: type A—linear molecules as nisin, subtilin, and epidermin, of which nisin is best characterized; and type B—globular molecules as mersacidin and mutacin.

Class II: consists thermostable low molecular peptides (<10 kDa) with 30–60 amino acid residues and unmodified nonlanthionine. Bacteriocins of this class do not undergo posttranslational modification. Three subdivisions have been proposed for this class. Class IIa consists of pedicine-like bacteriocins that have high specificity against *Listeria monocytogenes*. This includes leucocin mesentericin A and Y105, with 37 aa, and carnobacteriocin B2, with 48 aa. Class IIb requires the combination of two different peptides for bacteriocin activity since they cannot manifest antibacterial activity separately. Members of this group are lactacin F and lactococcin G. The bacteriocins belonging to class IIc have a covalent bond between C and N terminals, resulting in a cyclic structure, and are represented by enterocin AS48, circularin A and reutericin 6.

Class III: consists thermolabile bacteriocins of high molecular weight (>30 kDa), complex in nature of activity and protein structure. Its mechanism of action is distinct from other bacteriocins since they promote the lysis of the cell wall in sensitive cells and therefore can receive another name, bacteriolysins. They have an N-terminal domain homologous to endopeptidase and a C-terminal domain responsible for recognition by the sensitive cell. Lactacin A and B, helveticin J and V-1829, and acidophilucin A are examples of this group.

Class IV: According to Klaenhammer [14], this class consists of complex structures containing amino acids, carbohydrates, or lipids in its composition. However, this class is not recognized by other authors [6, 15] since they were not properly purified. Information related to this class is very limited.

Cotter et al. [16] proposed a new classification, wherein bacteriocins are divided into two categories: lantibiotics (class I) and nonlantibiotics (class II), while the high molecular proteins, consisting of class III, should receive a separate designation of "bacteriolisins." The authors also suggest the extinction of class IV. Because of their great biochemical diversity, the classification of bacteriocins is still under debate, and different classifications have been suggested over the years [4].

Bacteriocin is found to have bactericidal/bacteriostatic action and is affected by various factors, including dose, level of purity, indicator/pathogenic microbes physiological conditions, and environmental factors [9]. The antibacterial effect of bacteriocins generally relies on the pore formation, despite the differences between the several types of bacteriocin. There are a variety of modes of actions to attack the target bacteria, and a single bacteriocin can possess more than one mode of action [10]. The main mode of action against target cells involves the association with membrane lipids, leading to the formation of pores [4]. Pore formation results in changes of membrane permeability, with efflux of small metabolites (e.g., ions K^+, H^+, phosphate) of the susceptible cells, leading to the destruction of electrochemical gradient, leakage of cell contents, and cell death.

Because of their narrow target spectrum and high potencies, it is believed that most bacteriocins bind specific receptors on sensitive cells. A few of such bacteriocin receptors have indeed been identified, including mannose-phosphotransferase systems (man-PTS) and lipid II [4, 17]. The man-PTS is target by class IIa bacteriocins (e.g., pediocin PA-1, enterocin P, enterocin A and sakacin P) on sensitive cells of genera such as *Listeria*, *Enterococcus*, and *Lactobacillus* [4, 17].

Some lantibiotics (class I bacteriocins) use the cell wall precursor molecule lipid II as an anchoring receptor on target cells [17]. As the role of lipid II is common in all bacteria, these lantibiotics have a relatively broad inhibitory spectrum, including a number of different genera of Gram-positive bacteria [4].

While the antibacterial activity of bacteriocins is somewhat deciphered, their antiviral activity remains to be understood [18].

Due to their protein nature, all bacteriocins are inactivated by one or more proteolytic enzymes, including pancreatic (α-chymotrypsin and trypsin) and gastric origin (pepsin) [19], being generally harmless to the human body and surrounding environment [5]. This feature is very interesting for their use in food products.

Because of their high potency and specificity, bacteriocins are considered as promising antimicrobial agents for different applications, including food preservation and infection treatment [4, 13], especially the ones produced by acid lactic bacteria species (Gram-positive) [20]. Pure or mixed cultures of bacteriocin-producer lactic acid bacteria and bacteriocin produced by them can be used as protective system against common food spoilage bacteria and pathogens [9].

Bacteriocins can be used in three ways in food: (i) inoculating the food with lactic acid bacteria strains producing bacteriocins, (ii) the addition of purified or semipurified bacteriocin, and (iii) adding a fermented ingredient with strains of bacteriocinogenic [7]. Bacteriocin produced lactic acid bacteria used as start or coculture in food production can increase flavor and shelf-life [5]. Bacteriocins can also be used for those products that cannot be sterilized by thermal treatment, and even at freshly cut vegetables, fruits, and seed sprouts, which are consumed without cooking, this may lead to various health risk due to their contamination with pathogenic bacteria [9].

To preserve and stabilize various kinds of food, including fermented dairy products, mayonnaise-type spreads, cream, cheese products, and meat or vegetable compositions, whey from nisin-producing cultures is well documented [9]. Although many other type of bacteriocin such as subtilin, cerein, thuricin, plantaricin, etc., have been isolated and characterized from different bacteriocin producing strains of bacteria yet, to date the only commercially produced bacteriocins are nisin (*Lactococcus lactis*) and pediocin (*Pediococcus acidilactici*), and others are still in a process of getting commercial status to be used as food preservatives [9]

Since nisin is the most intensively studied and used bacteriocin, we present it in more detail in the following section.

2. Nisin

Nisin is a class I bacteriocin widely exploited and applied [13, 16, 21]. Initially, nisin was sold in England in 1953, and on the following decades, it was approved for use in over 48 countries. Nisin was considered safe for use in foods in 1969 by the Joint of Food and Agriculture Organization from World Health Organization (FAO/WHO) Expert Committee on Food Additives. In 1983, nisin was added in the European list of food additives under the number E234, and in 1988, it was approved by the US Food and Drug Agency (FDA) as generally regarded as safe (GRAS) for use in pasteurized products and processed cheeses to inhibit the growth of *Clostridium botulinum*.

Produced by species of *Lactococcus lactis* subsp. *Lactis*, nisin consists of 34 amino acid residues, with molecular weight of 3.5 kDa, and isoleucine (NH_2) and lysine (COOH) as terminal amino acids (Figure 1).

Nisin is ribosomally synthesized as a 57 amino acid peptide precursor, with 23 residues in the leader region and 34 residues in the framework region. Subsequently, through enzyme postmodification translocation, the leading region is removed; the serine and the threonine from the framework region undergo dehydration, resulting in the formation of dehydroalanine (Dha) and dehydrobutirine (Dhb), respectively. The subsequent reactions of cysteine sulfhydryl side chain with Dha and Dhb result in lanthionine thioether ring structures (Ala-S-Ala) and methyl-lanthionine (Aba-S-Aba). Finally, the active nisin is secreted and released by proteolytic cleavage of the leader peptide (23 amino acids) [20, 22].

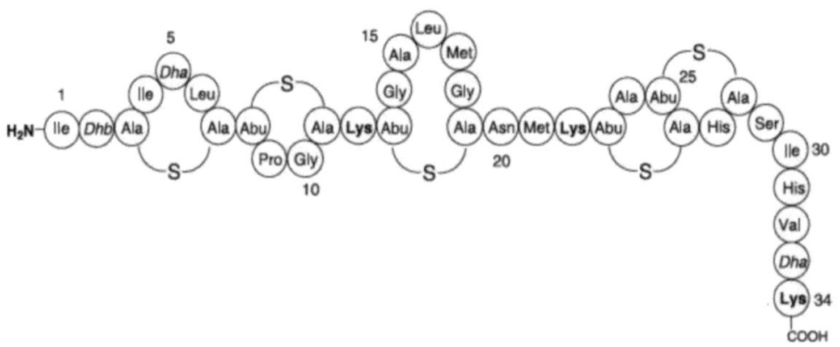

Figure 1. Schematic representation of the primary structure of nisin produced by *L. lactis* subsp. *lactis* ATCC 11454. Ala-Ala-S represents lanthionine; Abu-S-Ala-β-methyl, lanthionine, dehydroalanine Dha, and Dhb dehydrobutirine [19].

Nisin has in its composition amino acid rarely found in nature, such as dehydroalanine (Dha —02 residues), dehydrobutirine (Dhb—01 residue), lanthionine (Lan—01 residue), and methyl-lanthionine (Melan—04 residues), which can be responsible for important functional properties, as thermostability and bactericidal action [23]. Its cationic character is due to a combination of three lysine residues and one or more histidine residues [24]. Nisin is also an amphipathic molecule due to the presence of hydrophobic residues at the N-terminal region and the C-terminal hydrophilic region [19].

A natural nisin variant produced by *L. lactis* subsp. *lactis* ATCC 11454 is called nisin A and differs from nisin Z, produced by other species of *L. lactis,* by the change of the amino acid residue position 27, histidine in the nisin A to asparagines in nisin Z [25]. This substitution does not affect the antimicrobial activity but results in better properties of diffusion in the nisin Z [26]. The solubility of nisin Z is better than nisin A at a pH above 6 since the asparagine side chain is more polar than the one from histidine [27].

Nisin solubility, stability, and biological activity are highly dependent on pH, temperature, and nature of the substrate. The solubility and stability of nisin increase with increasing acidity. Thus, under neutral or alkaline conditions, nisin is almost insoluble. It is stable at thermal treatment and can be autoclaved at 121°C for 15 minutes, at pH 2–3 without denaturation and with an activity loss below 10% [28].

2.1. Mechanism of action, action spectrum, and toxicity effects

Nisin has antimicrobial effect against a broad spectrum of Gram-positive bacteria and spore germination but shows little or no activity on Gram-negative bacteria, fungi, or viruses. Both vegetative cells and spores are sensitive to nisin, but the spores are usually more sensitive than the vegetative form. Depending on its concentration, nisin can be bactericidal or bacteriostatic [29]

Nisin has demonstrated antibacterial activity against pathogenic bacteria such as *Streptococcus mutans, Streptococcus sanguinis, Lactobacillus acidophilus,* and *Enterococcus faecalis* and is highly active against *Listeria monocytogenes, Staphylococcus aureus, Bacillus cereus, Lactobacillus plantarum, Micrococcus luteus,* and *Micrococcus flavus* [21, 30, 31].

Nisin acts by a dual mode of action, combining both the mechanisms: pore formation, and in the vegetative cells, it interferes in the cell wall synthesis. Since it is positively charged with hydrophobic parts, electrostatic interactions with the phosphate group negatively charged from the cell membrane occur, leading to nisin connection with the target cell. Here, lipid II serves as a docking molecule and mediates a "targeted" pore formation [32]. The formation of pores in the membrane with 2–2.5 nm in diameter allows small and essential molecules (K^+, ATP, and amino acids) to leak from the cell, resulting in the disruption of the barrier function and, consequently, in the dissipation of the membrane potential. Finally, this results in the abrupt arrest of all cellular processes and in cell death [32] (Figure 2). The mechanism of forming pores is the same as the one used by other lantibiotics, as lacticin 3147, subtilin, and epidermin, among others.

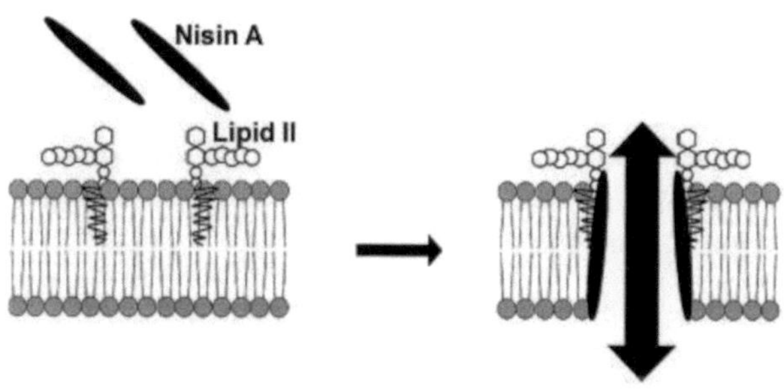

Figure 2. Nisin mode of action on a cell target. The nisin N-terminus binds to the lipid II, permeabilizes the membrane, and leads to pore formation [10].

Studies have shown that nisin also interferes with cell wall biosynthesis, by its ability to bind to lipid II, a peptidoglycan precursor, inhibiting then the cell wall biosynthesis [6, 33–36]. The N-terminal rings (A and B) form a binding pocket, the pyrophosphate cage that allows binding to the pyrophosphate moiety of lipid I/II. Complex formation with lipid II prevents transglycosylation by steric hindrance and results in the sequestration of the precursors and, hence, in its abduction from the sites of nascent cell wall biosynthesis[32].

In Gram-negative bacteria, the outer layer composed of lipopolysaccharide (LPS) acts as a barrier to the nisin action on the cytoplasmic wall. However, the addition of chelating agents, such as EDTA, confines the Mg^{2+} and Ca^{+} from LPS and destabilizes the LPS layer. Therefore, nisin can be transported through the LPS layer and create pores in the cytoplasmic membrane, causing the loss of the proton motive force and intracellular nutrients [37].

The mechanism by which nisin prevents the germination of spores is different from the one that occurs in the vegetative cells. It is believed that the dehydroalanine residue (Dha) in the 5-position interacts with vital sulfhydryl groups present on the membrane of freshly germinated spores and exert a profound bacteriostatic effect, resulting in subsequent inhibition of spore. Thus, nisin allows the germination of spores but inhibits subsequent steps of the new cell formation process [38, 39]

Toxicology studies have shown that nisin intake does not cause toxic effects to the human body, and LD50 reported was 6950 mg/kg, similar to table salt, when administered orally [40]. Research conducted in the oral microflora showed that 1 minute after consuming chocolate containing nisin, only 1/40 of the original nisin activity was detected in saliva [6]. Nisin could cause hemolysis at concentrations that were 1000-fold higher than those required for antimicrobial activity [41].

Based on the "no effect" level observed in toxicological evaluations of animals and allowed for humans, the WHO recommends as the Acceptable Daily Intake (ADI, maximum amount of additive that could be ingested daily without causing any damage to consumer health) of 33,000 international units (IU) (0.825 mg) per kilogram of body weight [21].

Despite the wide application of nisin as natural food preservative, especially in dairy products, there is no agreement on the maximum levels allowed between countries where its use was legally approved, e.g., nisin can be added to cheese without limit in the UK [42].

2.2. Production and purification

Nisin production is affected by many factors such as the producer species, composition of the culture medium, pH, temperature, agitation, aeration, adsorption of nisin by the producing cells, and enzymatic degradation [43].

The release of nisin from the cells to the medium is pH dependent. At pH lower than 6, more than 80% of the produced nisin is extracellularly released. At pH higher than 6, most of nisin produced is associated to the cell membrane or intracellularly [44]. Nisin can also be reversibly adsorbed by some proteins or by the producer cell. In general, between 93% and 100% of bacteriocins are adsorbed at pH near 6.0, and the lower adsorption ($\leq 5\%$) is around pH 1.5 to 2.0. They are also highly sensitive to the action of proteolytic enzymes [6, 45].

At laboratory scale, commercial culture media is used, such as MRS and M17 broth, but their high cost makes them impractical for large-scale production. In addition, the culture medium usually contains excess of protein (tryptone, peptone, meat extract, and yeast extract), leading to the nonconsumption of a substantial proportion and unnecessary costs and difficulties to

http://dx.doi.org/10.5772/60932

the nisin purification processes [46]. The components cost from the culture medium may vary between 38% and 73% of the total production cost, and the carbon source is the most expensive item from the medium [47].

In this sense, industrial wastes have aroused the interest to be used as raw material for bacteriocins production. Whey, a milk byproduct, discarded by the dairy industry, has been used in some researches for the production of nisin [48, 49].

Mondragón-Parada and coworkers [50] supplemented whey with minerals and small amounts of yeast extract in order to obtain lactic acid bacteria biomass production. Liu and collaborators [51] also studied a whey supplemented medium to obtain simultaneous nisin and lactic acid. Lactic acid is used in the food industry and in the production of poly lactic acid, a biodegradable biopolymer. However, the small amount of lactic acid obtained by these authors became the separation process expensive.

Commercial media, different combinations of commercials substrates at low concentrations, milk, and milk whey have been tested at microaerophilic conditions for the production of enterocin EJ97 bacteriocin. The highest bacteriocin activity was obtained using pasteurized buffered milk whey as growth substrate [52].

Penna and coworkers [53] conducted studies where shaker cultures of *L. lactis* with media containing 25% milk and 25% MRS or M17 broth were satisfactory for producing nisin.

Bioengineering techniques to improve bacteriocins production have been studied by some authors [54–57]. They report a greater production of nisin by genetically modified strains. Moreover, these techniques could improve antimicrobial activity of nisin or its stability at elevated temperature and/or under neutral or alkaline conditions.

The semipurified nisin preparations are processed by food-grade techniques. An example is Nisaplin™, a commercial preparation obtained from the fermentation of *L. lactis* on milk medium. The fermented resultant is subsequently concentrated, separated, processed by spray dryer technique, and turned into small particles. The final product consists of 2.5% of nisin contained in NaCl and denatured milk solids [58]. The amount of 1 g of this product is standardized with an activity of 10^6 IU.

Specific purification protocols were designed for nisin purification depending on its final usage (e.g., food, drug, cosmetics). Nisin has been purified using expanded bed ion exchange chromatography [59], immune-affinity chromatography [60, 61], ion exchange chromatography, hydrophobic interaction chromatography, gel filtration, and reversed-phase high-pressure liquid chromatography [62, 63]. There are also some nisin extraction protocols, using organic solvents, such as ethanol and methanol [64], or ammonium sulfate precipitation and acid precipitation (pH 2.0) [65].

Nisin is highly active in acid pH but lose activity above pH 7. It is not effective for meat preservation due to the presence of components, such as phospholipids, which limit nisin activity. High-fat content also can affect uniform distribution of nisin in food [58]. A moderate concentration of NaCl, present in many foods, is responsible for neutralizing nisin action [66]. Food additives such as sodium metabisulfite (an antioxidant) and titanium dioxide (a colorant) are frequently used in food and also affect the antimicrobial activity of nisin [67]. Nisin activity efficiency could also be affect by the contamination level of the food [20].

2.3. Nisin application

Nisin is applied as natural preservative in food, such as cheese, butter, canned, alcoholic drinks, sausages, pasteurized liquid egg, and salad dressings, among others [67], alone or in combination with other conservation methods. Other applications in preservation technologies include the development of antimicrobial active packaging [68], liposomes [69], and nanodelivery systems [70].

Although the main application of nisin is in foods, particularly dairy products, research have found its potential for therapeutic purposes, such as treatment of atopic dermatitis [71], stomach ulcers, and colon intestinal infections for patients with immunodeficiency [72, 73]. Researchers have shown the effectiveness of the antimicrobial activity of nisin in control of respiratory tract infections caused by *S. aureus* in an animal model [74]. Fernández and coworkers [75] studied the use of nisin as an efficient alternative to antibiotics for the treatment of staphylococcal mastitis in women during lactation.

Aranha et al. [76] studied the nisin application as vaginal contraceptive for humans. Gupta et al. [77] continued the research and showed no toxicity evidence for nisin has, suggesting its potential clinical application as a prophylactic vaginal contraceptive for women. Nisin has also been evaluated for use in toothpaste [78]. Others examples of nisin application are describe in Table 2.

Area	Application	Studies
Endodontic	Dental caries treatment and root canal infection	[31]
Food control	Oil emulsions, cheese preservative	[79, 80]
Nanotechnology	Coated antibiolfim, food biopreservative	[70, 81]
Pharmaceutical industry	Herpes treatment, respiratory tract infection	[3, 74]
Veterinary	Mastitis	[82]

Table 2. Examples of nisin applications.

Nisin represents an advance for the microbiological safety in dairy products. Further, research is needed to identify drawbacks that may affect their future applications, as the development of innovative in the pharmaceutical, nanotechnological, and medical areas.

3. Conclusion

Increased interest has been shown in antimicrobial peptides (AMPs), especially as an alternative to antibiotics. However, because many AMPs are toxic to mammalian cells, they are not good candidates for therapies [83]. Bacteriocins, AMPs produced by bacteria, have shown little or no toxicity to humans, especially the ones produced by lactic acid bacteria (LAB). Bacteriocins possess vast potential as additive or as substitute for existing antimicrobial compounds, which can be used in formulation of different food products [9].

The most studied and interest bacteriocin from LAB is nisin, which is currently used in over 50 countries as a food preservative. Nisin holds many characteristics and chemical properties, like low molecular weight, thermal stability, lack of toxicity, low tendency to generate resistance, and low immunogenicity, which make it suitable for potential applications in different health care associated settings such as in human and veterinary medicine and in biochemical, pharmaceutical, agricultural, or food industries [32]. Nisin has been employed as a biological food preservative in processed dairy products, canned fruits, and vegetables for more than 50 years [32]. The potential of bacteriocins as promising alternatives for traditional antimicrobial therapeutics, as probiotics or preservatives in different areas of the healthcare sector and in associated industries, has been discussed for many years. So far, only nisin has been successfully introduced as a preservative into food industry or as a prophylactic in veterinary settings [32]. Moreover, nisin has a potential role for a new product that is cost-competitive and also provides high quality for them, especially for products having strict specifications of safety and quality supervision.

Acknowledgements

This research was supported by grants from CAPES (Coordenação de Aperfeiçoamento de Pessoal de Nível Superior, Brazil), CNPq (Conselho Nacional de Desenvolvimento Científico e Tecnológico, Brazil), and FAPESP (Fundação de Amparo à Pesquisa do Estado de São Paulo, Brazil).

Author details

Angela Faustino Jozala[1], Letícia Celia de Lencastre Novaes[2] and Adalberto Pessoa Junior[3*]

*Address all correspondence to: pessoajr@usp.br

1 Department of Pharmacy, School of Pharmacy, Sorocaba University–UNISO, Sorocaba, SP, Brazil

2 Department of Clinical Pathology, Faculty of Medical Sciences, University of Campinas, Campinas, Brazil

3 Department of Biochemical and Pharmaceutical Technology, School of Pharmaceutical Science University of São Paulo, São Paulo, Brazil

References

[1] Izadpanah A, Gallo RL (2005). Antimicrobial peptides. J Am Acad Dermatol 52:381–90; quiz 391–2.

[2] Guaní-Guerra E, Santos-Mendoza T, Lugo-Reyes SO, Terán LM (2010). Antimicrobial peptides: general overview and clinical implications in human health and disease. Clin Immunol 135:1–11.

[3] Reddy KVR, Yedery RD, Aranha C (2004). Antimicrobial peptides: premises and promises. Int J Antimicrob Agents 24:536–547.

[4] Hassan M, Kjos M, Nes IF, Diep DB, Lotfipour F (2012). Natural antimicrobial peptides from bacteria: characteristics and potential applications to fight against antibiotic resistance. J Appl Microbiol 113:723–36.

[5] Yang S-C, Lin C-H, Sung CT, Fang J-Y (2014). Antibacterial activities of bacteriocins: application in foods and pharmaceuticals. Front Microbiol 5:241.

[6] Cleveland J, Montville TJ, Nes IF, Chikindas ML (2001). Bacteriocins: safe, natural antimicrobials for food preservation. Int J Food Microbiol 71:1–20.

[7] Barbosa MS (2009). Avaliação da ação de ingredientes da matriz alimentar na atividade antilisteria das bacteriocinas produzidas por Lactobacillus sakei subsp. sakei 2a. 95.

[8] Todorov SD, Dicks LMT (2009). Effect of modified MRS medium on production and purification of antimicrobial peptide ST4SA produced by *Enterococcus mundtii*. Anaerobe 15:65–73.

[9] Bali V, Panesar PS, Bera MB, Kennedy JF (2014). Bacteriocins: recent trends and potential applications. Crit Rev Food Sci Nutr 140813060811009.

[10] Nishie M, Nagao J-I, Sonomoto K (2012). Antibacterial peptides "bacteriocins": an overview of their diverse characteristics and applications. Biocontrol Sci 17:1–16.

[11] Karpiński TM, Szkaradkiewicz AK (2013). Characteristic of bacteriocines and their application. Polish J Microbiol 62:223–235.

[12] De Vuyst L, Leroy F (2007). Bacteriocins from lactic acid bacteria: production, purification, and food applications. J Mol Microbiol Biotechnol 13:194–199.

[13] Zacharof MP, Lovitt RW (2012). Bacteriocins produced by lactic acid bacteria a review article. APCBEE Procedia 2:50–56.

[14] Klaenhammer TR (1993). Genetics of bacteriocins produced by lactic-acid bacteria. Fems Microbiol Rev 12:39–86.

[15] Savadogo A, Ouattara CAT, Bassole IHN, Traore SA (2006). Bacteriocins and lactic acid bacteria—a minireview. African J Biotechnol 5:678–683.

[16] Cotter PD, Hill C, Ross RP (2005). Bacteriocins: developing innate immunity for food. Nat Rev Microbiol 3:777–788.

[17] Hammami R, Fernandez B, Lacroix C, Fliss I (2013).. Anti-infective properties of bacteriocins: an update. Cell Mol Life Sci 70:2947–2967.

[18] Al Kassaa I, Hober D, Hamze M, Chihib NE, Drider D (2014). Antiviral potential of lactic acid bacteria and their bacteriocins. Probiotics Antimicrob Proteins 6:177–185.

[19] De Vuyst L, Vandamme EJ (1994). Bacteriocins of lactic acid bacteria microbiology, genetics and applications. doi: 10.1007/978-1-4615-2668-1.

[20] Balciunas EM, Castillo Martinez FA, Todorov SD, Franco BDGDM, Converti A, Oliveira RPDS (2013). Novel biotechnological applications of bacteriocins: a review. Food Control 32:134–142.

[21] De Arauz LJ, Jozala AF, Mazzola PG, Vessoni Penna TC (2009). Nisin biotechnological production and application: a review. Trends Food Sci Technol 20:146–154.

[22] Sonomoto K, Chinachoti N, Endo N, Ishizaki A (2000). Biosynthetic production of nisin Z by immobilized *Lactococcus lactis* IO-1. J Mol Catal B Enzym 10:325–334.

[23] De Vuyst L, Vandamme EJ (1992). Influence of the carbon source on nisin production in *Lactococcus lactis* subsp. lactis batch fermentations. J Gen Microbiol 138:571–578.

[24] Bhatti M, Veeramachaneni A, Shelef LA (2004). Factors affecting the antilisterial effects of nisin in milk. Int J Food Microbiol 97:215–219.

[25] Benech RO, Kheadr EE, Lacroix C, Fliss I (2002). Antibacterial activities of nisin Z encapsulated in liposomes or produced in situ by mixed culture during Cheddar cheese ripening. Appl Environ Microbiol 68:5607–5619.

[26] Laridi R, Kheadr EE, Benech RO, Vuillemard JC, Lacroix C, Fliss I (2003). Liposome encapsulated nisin Z: optimization, stability and release during milk fermentation. Int Dairy J 13:325–336.

[27] Matsusaki H, Endo N, Sonomoto K, Ishizaki A (1996). Lantibiotic nisin Z fermentative production by *Lactococcus lactis* IO-1: relationship between production of the lantibiotic and lactate and cell growth. Appl Microbiol Biotechnol 45:36–40.

[28] Delves-Broughton J (1990). Nisin and its application as a food preservative. J Soc Dairy Technol 43:73–76.

[29] Tsukiyama RI, Katsura H, Tokuriki N, Kobayashi M (2002). Antibacterial activity of licochalcone A against spore-forming bacteria. Antimicrob Agents Chemother 46:1226–1230.

[30] Rilla N, Martínez B, Rodríguez A (2004). Inhibition of a methicillin-resistant *Staphylococcus aureus* strain in Afuega'l Pitu cheese by the nisin Z-producing strain *Lactococcus lactis* subsp. lactis IPLA 729. J Food Prot 67:928–933.

[31] Tong Z, Ni L, Ling J (2014). Antibacterial peptide nisin: a potential role in the inhibition of oral pathogenic bacteria. Peptides 60:32–40.

[32] Dischinger J, Basi Chipalu S, Bierbaum G (2014). Lantibiotics: promising candidates for future applications in health care. Int J Med Microbiol 304:51–62.

[33] Von Staszewski M, Jagus RJ (2008). Natural antimicrobials: effect of Microgard and nisin against *Listeria innocua* in liquid cheese whey. Int Dairy J 18:255–259.

[34] Breukink E, de Kruijff B (2006). Lipid II as a target for antibiotics. Nat Rev Drug Discov 5:321–332.

[35] Breukink E, Van Heusden HE, Vollmerhaus PJ, Swiezewska E, Brunner L, Walker S, Heck AJR, De Kruijff B (2003). Lipid II is an intrinsic component of the pore induced by nisin in bacterial membranes. J Biol Chem 278:19898–19903.

[36] Hasper HE, De Kruijff B, Breukink E (2004). Assembly and stability of nisin-Lipid II pores. Biochemistry 43:11567–11575.

[37] Millette M, Smoragiewicz W, Lacroix M (2004). Antimicrobial potential of immobilized *Lactococcus lactis* subsp. lactis ATCC 11454 against selected bacteria. J Food Prot 67:1184–1189.

[38] Asaduzzaman SM, Sonomoto K (2009). Lantibiotics: diverse activities and unique modes of action. J Biosci Bioeng 107:475–487.

[39] Gut IM, Blanke SR, Van Der Donk WA (2011). Mechanism of inhibition of bacillus anthracis spore outgrowth by the Lantibiotic Nisin. ACS Chem Biol 6:744–752.

[40] Hoover DG, Steenson LR (1993). Bacteriocins of Lactic Acid Bacteria. Academic Press. 275 pp.

[41] Maher S, McClean S (2006). Investigation of the cytotoxicity of eukaryotic and prokaryotic antimicrobial peptides in intestinal epithelial cells in vitro. Biochem Pharmacol 71:1289–1298.

[42] Sobrino-López A, Martín-Belloso O (2008). Use of nisin and other bacteriocins for preservation of dairy products. Int Dairy J 18:329–343.

[43] Pongtharangku T, Demirci A (2007). Online recovery of nisin during fermentation and its effect on nisin production in biofilm reactor. Appl Microbiol Biotechnol 74:555–562.

[44] Penna TCV, Jozala AF, Gentille TR, Pessoa Júnior A, Cholewa O (2006). Detection of nisin expression by *Lactococcus lactis* using two susceptible bacteria to associate the effects of nisin with EDTA. Appl Biochem Biotechnol 129-132:334–346.

[45] Yang R, Ray B (1994). Factors influencing production of bacteriocins by lactic acid bacteria. Food Microbiol 11:281–291.

[46] Vázquez JA, González MP, Murado MA (2006). Preliminary tests on nisin and pediocin production using waste protein sources: factorial and kinetic studies. Bioresour Technol 97:605–613.

[47] Schmidell W, Lima UA, Aquarone E, Borzani W (2001). Biotecnologia industrial. São Paulo: Ed. Edgard Blücher Ltda. 541 pp.

[48] Guerra NP, Rua ML, Pastrana L (2001). Nutritional factors affecting the production of two bacteriocins from lactic acid bacteria on whey. Int J Food Microbiol 70:267–281.

[49] De Arauz LJ, Jozala AF, Pinheiro GS, Mazzola PG, Pessoa A, Penna TC V (2008). Nisin expression production from *Lactococcus lactis* in milk whey medium. J Chem Technol Biotechnol 83:325–328.

[50] Mondragón-Parada ME, Nájera-Martínez M, Juárez-Ramírez C, Galíndez-Mayer J, Ruiz-Ordaz N, Cristiani-Urbina E (2006). Lactic acid bacteria production from whey. Appl Biochem Biotechnol 134:223–232.

[51] Liu C, Liu Y, Liao W, Wen Z, Chen S (2004). Simultaneous production of nisin and lactic acid from cheese whey: optimization of fermentation conditions through statistically based experimental designs. Appl Biochem Biotechnol 113–116:627–638.

[52] López RL, García MT, Abriouel H, Omar N Ben, Grande MJ, Martínez-Cañamero M, Gálvez A (2007). Semi-preparative scale purification of enterococcal bacteriocin enterocin EJ97, and evaluation of substrates for its production. J Ind Microbiol Biotechnol 34:779–785.

[53] Penna TCV, Jozala AF, De Lencastre Novaes LC, Pessoa A, Cholewa O (2005). Production of nisin by *Lactococcus lactis* in media with skimmed milk. Appl Biochem Biotechnol 121–124:619–637.

[54] Suda S, Westerbeek A, O'Connor PM, Ross RP, Hill C, Cotter PD (2010). Effect of bioengineering lacticin 3147 lanthionine bridges on specific activity and resistance to heat and proteases. Chem Biol 17:1151–1160.

[55] Collins B, Cotter PD, Hill C, Ross RP (2010). Applications of lactic acid bacteria-produced bacteriocins. Biotechnol Lact Acid Bact Nov Appl. 89–109.

[56] Chen P, Novak J, Kirk M, Barnes S, Qi F, Caufield PW (1998). Structure-activity study of the lantibiotic mutacin II from *Streptococcus mutans* T8 by a gene replacement strategy. Appl Environ Microbiol 64:2335–2340.

[57] Yuan J, Zhang ZZ, Chen XZ, Yang W, Huan LD (2004). Site-directed mutagenesis of the hinge region of nisinZ and properties of nisinZ mutants. Appl Microbiol Biotechnol 64:806–815.

[58] Deegan LH, Cotter PD, Hill C, Ross P (2006). Bacteriocins: biological tools for biopreservation and shelf-life extension. Int Dairy J 16:1058–1071.

[59] Cheigh CI, Kook MC, Kim SB, Hong YH, Pyun YR (2004). Simple one-step purification of nisin Z from unclarified culture broth of *Lactococcus lactis* subsp. lactis A164 using expanded bed ion exchange chromatography. Biotechnol Lett 26:1341–1345.

[60] Prioult G, Turcotte C, Labarre L, Lacroix C, Fliss I (2000). Rapid purification of nisin Z using specific monoclonal antibody-coated magnetic beads. Int Dairy J 10:627–633.

[61] Suárez AM, Azcona JI, Rodríguez JM, Sanz B, Hernández PE (1997). One-step purification of nisin A by immunoaffinity chromatography. Appl Environ Microbiol 63:4990–4992.

[62] Saavedra L, Castellano P, Sesma F (2004). Purification of bacteriocins produced by lactic acid bacteria. Methods Mol Biol 268:331–336.

[63] Garsa AK, Kumariya R, Sood SK, Kumar A, Kapila S (2014). Bacteriocin production and different strategies for their recovery and purification. Probiotics Antimicrob Proteins 6:47–58.

[64] Xiao D, Michael Davidson P, D'Souza DH, Lin J, Zhong Q (2010). Nisin extraction capacity of aqueous ethanol and methanol from a 2.5% preparation. J Food Eng 100:194–200.

[65] Yang R, Johnson MC, Ray B (1992). Novel method to extract large amounts of bacteriocins from lactic acid bacteria. Appl Environ Microbiol 58:3355–3359.

[66] Devlieghere F, Vermeiren L, Debevere J (2004). New preservation technologies: possibilities and limitations. Int Dairy J. 273–285.

[67] Delves-Broughton J (1996). Applications of the bacteriocin, nisin. Antonie van Leeuwenhoek, Int J Gen Mol Microbiol 69:193–202.

[68] Lucera A, Costa C, Conte A, Del Nobile MA (2012). Food applications of natural antimicrobial compounds. Front Microbiol. doi: 10.3389/fmicb.2012.00287.

[69] Malheiros P da S, Sant'Anna V, Barbosa M de S, Brandelli A, Franco BDG de M (2012). Effect of liposome-encapsulated nisin and bacteriocin-like substance P34 on *Listeria monocytogenes* growth in Minas frescal cheese. Int J Food Microbiol 156:272–277.

[70] Imran M, Revol-Junelles A-M, Paris C, Guedon E, Linder M, Desobry S (2015) Liposomal nanodelivery systems using soy and marine lecithin to encapsulate food biopreservative nisin. LWT—Food Sci Technol. doi: 10.1016/j.lwt.2014.12.046.

[71] Valenta C, Bernkop-Schnürch A, Rigler HP (1996). The antistaphylococcal effect of nisin in a suitable vehicle: a potential therapy for atopic dermatitis in man. J Pharm Pharmacol 48:988–991.

[72] Dubois A (1995). Spiral bacteria in the human stomach: the gastric helicobacters. Emerg Infect Dis 1:79–85.

[73] Sakamoto I, Igarashi M, Kimura K, Takagi A, Miwa T, Koga Y (2001). Suppressive effect of *Lactobacillus gasseri* OLL 2716 (LG21) on *Helicobacter pylori* infection in humans. J Antimicrob Chemother 47:709–710.

[74] De Kwaadsteniet M, Doeschate KT, Dicks LMT (2009). Nisin F in the treatment of respiratory tract infections caused by *Staphylococcus aureus*. Lett Appl Microbiol 48:65–70.

[75] Fernández L, Delgado S, Herrero H, Maldonado A, Rodríguez JM (2008). The bacteriocin nisin, an effective agent for the treatment of staphylococcal mastitis during lactation. J Hum Lact 24:311–316.

[76] Aranha C, Gupta S, Reddy KVR (2004). Contraceptive efficacy of antimicrobial peptide nisin: in vitro and in vivo studies. Contraception 69:333–338.

[77] Gupta SM, Aranha CC, Reddy KVR (2008). Evaluation of developmental toxicity of microbicide Nisin in rats. Food Chem Toxicol 46:598–603.

[78] Kim WS, Hall RJ, Dunn NW (1997). The effect of nisin concentration and nntrient depletion on nisin production of *Lactococcus lactis*. Appl Microbiol Biotechnol 48:449–453.

[79] Chen H, Davidson PM, Zhong Q (2014). Antimicrobial properties of nisin after glycation with lactose, maltodextrin and dextran and the thyme oil emulsions prepared thereof. Int J Food Microbiol 191:75–81.

[80] Chollet E, Sebti I, Martial-Gros A, Degraeve P (2008). Nisin preliminary study as a potential preservative for sliced ripened cheese: NaCl, fat and enzymes influence on nisin concentration and its antimicrobial activity. Food Control 19:982–989.

[81] Dong X, McCoy E, Zhang M, Yang L (2014). Inhibitory effects of nisin-coated multiwalled carbon nanotube sheet on biofilm formation from *Bacillus anthracis* spores. J Environ Sci 26:2526–2534.

[82] Cao LT, Wu JQ, Xie F, Hu SH, Mo Y (2007). Efficacy of nisin in treatment of clinical mastitis in lactating dairy cows. J Dairy Sci 90:3980–3985.

[83] Allen HK, Trachsel J, Looft T, Casey TA (2014). Finding alternatives to antibiotics. Ann N Y Acad Sci 1323:1–10.

Section 3

The Alternatives

Chapter 6

Natural Products as Antibacterial Agents — Antibacterial Potential and Safety of Post-distillation and Waste Material from *Thymus vulgaris* L., Lamiaceae

Neda Gavarić, Jasna Kovač, Nadine Kretschmer,
Nebojša Kladar, Sonja Smole Možina, Franz Bucar,
Rudolf Bauer and Biljana Božin

Additional information is available at the end of the chapter

http://dx.doi.org/10.5772/60869

Abstract

Medicinal plants have a long tradition of use in folk and conventional medicine. In recent years numerous studies confirm various bioactivities of natural products, among them antibacterial activity. Natural antibacterial agents such are essential oils and isolated compounds now represent a notable source for pharmaceutical and food industry and are widely used in cosmetology. They meet standards of 'green consumerism' together with excellent antibacterial activity. Aromatic plants such is *Thymus vulgaris* L. are the major sources of essential oils. Thyme essential oil, as well as dominant compounds thymol and carvacrol are generally recognised as safe and have been registered by European Commission for use as flavouring agents in foodstuffs. However, essential oil is present in very low amount (0,8-2,6%) in thyme leaves. Thus, the majority of plant material remains unused after the isolation. Nowadays, the biological potential of various plant waste materials are in focus of numerous studies. These investigations also include the antimicrobial activity considering the fact that waste material extracts represent the valuable source of different phenolic compounds. Regarding all this, the aim of the present study was to determine antibacterial potential of chemically characterised extracts obtained from waste material remaining after the preparation of drug (stems) and isolation of thyme essential oil (deodorised leaves, postdistillation decoction) on selected bacterial strains. Also, in order to determine safety of waste extracts their cytotoxicity was investigated. All extracts were prepared with maceration using 45% or 75% ethanol

(EtOH) for 24 h at room temperature (1:10 w/v). Total phenolic compounds and flavonoids were determined spectrophotometrically. Extracts were chemically characterized by HPLC/DAD analysis. Antibacerial testing was done with broth dilution method against several bacterial strains (*Staphylococcus aureus, Bacillus cereus, Salmonella infantis, Escherichia coli* and *Campylobacter jejuni*). Cytotoxicity and cytoprotection studies were performed by XTT assay. Result of HPLC analysis showed that investigated extracts, especially those obtained from deodorised leaves represent a valuable source of rosmarinic acid and luteolin 7-O-glucuronide. Antibacterial testing indicated that all waste material extracts, except the extract T2, possess similar or even stronger bacteriostatic activity than T1. No cytotoxicity nor cytoprotection were determined. In conclusion, results of this study confirmed antibacterial potential investigated thyme extracts. High concentrations of rosmarinic acid and luteolin 7-O-glucuronide, which both have numerous pharmacological activities, were determined. This indicates that thyme postdistillation waste material extracts could be used for isolation of dominant compounds or as addities in pharmaceutical and food industry.

Keywords: aromatic plants, thyme, postdistillation waste, antibacterial potential, cytotoxicity

1. Introduction

Plants have been used as food, spice, and medicine since ancient time. Much before the discovery of the existence of microorganisms, plants were an integrated part of the traditional medicine of many communities used for the treatment of various infectious diseases. Likewise, the use of plants as spices, not only affected the organoleptic properties of food, but it was also one of the ways for its preservation [1]. Today, modern consumers demand food that will be minimally processed and contain, as much as possible, additives of natural origin that unlike synthetic ones, will be safe and ecologically acceptable. Also, the approach in raising livestock and production of food of plant origin is shifting towards the use of traditional methods in protection against pests and diseases [2]. In addition, the irrational use of antibiotics not only in human and veterinary medicine, but also to promote growth in agriculture, has led to more frequent occurrence of resistance to conventional antibiotics of some pathogenic microorganisms [3, 4, 5] such are *Escherichia coli, Staphylococcus aureus, Enterococcus* spp., *Salmonella* spp., and *Campylobacter* spp. [6, 7, 8, 9]. Moreover, it is important to bear in mind the potential synergistic action of different natural products and conventional antibiotics in order to affect the emerging resistance [10, 11, 12].

Aromatic plants such as *Thymus vulgaris* L. (common thyme) and many other representatives of the family Lamiaceae have a long tradition of use in both folk and conventional medicine and in the pharmaceutical industry [13]. Common thyme is indigenous to Europe, especially the Mediterranean region, and is extensively cultivated worldwide. It is a small, bushy herb, with small, elliptical, greenish-grey, and shortly-stalked leaves. Thyme has a characteristic odour of thymol and is used as a culinary herb [14]. The active principle is the essential oil (*Thymi aetheroleum*), with thymol (25%–50%) and carvacrol (3%–10%) as dominant compounds (Table 1) (Figure 1) [15].

Compounds	Percentage (%)	References
Monoterpene Hydrocarbons		
α-Terpinene	1.25–3.17	17
p-Cimene	0.8–16.13	16, 17
γ-Terpinene	7.3–1.87	12, 16, 17
Oxygenated Monoterpenes		
1, 8-Cineole	0.8–2.17	16, 17
Linalool	2.03–6.8	12, 16, 17
Menthone	2.2	16
Borneol	2.6–8.9	12, 16
Neomenthol	2.8	16
Terpinen-4-ol	1–2.63	16, 17
Aromatic Oxygenated Monoterpenes		
Carvacrol methyl ether	3.9	12
Thymol	35.51–47.9	12, 16, 17
Carvacrol	4.43–12	
Sesquiterpene Hydrocarbons		
trans-Caryophyllene	1.13–5.1	12, 17
β-Cubebene	2.4	16
Oxygenated Sesquiterpenes		
Caryophyllene oxide	0.33–4.6	12, 17
Aliphatic compounds		
1-Octen-3-ol	2.8	12

Table 1. Dominant compounds of *Thymus vulgaris* essential oil

The percentage of the major constituents varies greatly, depending on numerous complex factors, both endogenous and exogenous such are: chemotype, ontogenesis, geographic and climatic conditions, methods used for plant material processing, and essential oil isolation [18]. Also, similar to other medicinal plants, the drug could be adulterated or replaced with other representatives of the genus *Thymus*, such as *T. serpyllum*, *T. marschallianus*, *T. pannonicus*, etc., that affect the differences in chemical composition and biological activities [19, 20]. Nevertheless, a minimum 40% of the thyme essential oil is required to be aromatic oxygenated monoterpenes [15].

	Thyme essential oil (µl/mL)	Thymol (µg/mL)	Carvacrol (µg/mL)	References
Staphylococcus aureus	0.2–2.5	250–2000	125–280	12, 21, 22
Salmonella sp.	0.45–20	250–3755	125–375	3, 12, 21
Escherichia coli	0.45–1.25	250–2000	125–560	12, 21, 22, 23
Bacillus cereus	1	250–560	125–140	12, 21

Table 2. Minimal inhibitory concentrations of thyme essential oil, thymol, and carvacrol on selected bacterial strains

Thyme essential oil, thymol, and carvacrol are generally recognised as safe (GRAS status) and have been registered by the European Commission for use as flavouring agents in foods [24]. GRAS is a rigorous process that relies on common knowledge and expert consensus about the safety of the substance for its intended use. Well-conducted toxicology studies are one of the factors that are used to assess the safety of various natural products, for example, plant extracts or essential oils that are composed of a mixture of tens or hundreds of compounds [25].

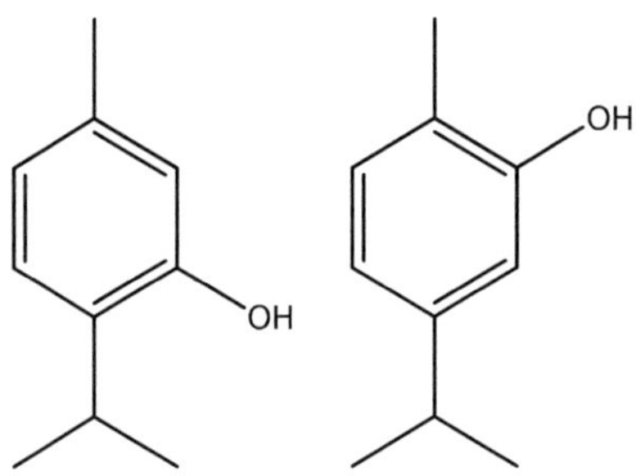

Figure 1. Chemical structures of dominant monoterpenes in thyme essential oil

In recent years, numerous studies confirm various bioactivities of thyme essential oil and isolated dominant monoterpenes, among them antibacterial and antifungal activity, together with the inhibition of mycotoxin production (Table 2) [3, 12, 16, 21, 23, 26, 27, 28]. Generally, most of the essential oils used in the pharmaceutical, cosmetic, and food industries possess strong antioxidant activity and represent a notable source of natural additives for different products [12, 29, 30]. What is more important is that they meet standards of 'green consumerism' [21]. However, the essential oil is present in very low amounts (0.8%–2.6%) in thyme leaves. Thus, the majority of plant material remains unused after the isolation.

On the other hand, thyme leaves are found to be a rich source of various phenolic compounds, particularly phenolic acids, flavonoids, and other secondary metabolites that are expected to contribute to its biological activities (Table 3) [14].

Rosmarinic acid is an ester of caffeic acid and 3,4-dihydroxyphenyllactic acid (Figure 5) widely found in the plant kingdom and presumably accumulated as a defense compound. In the

Lamiaceae family, the occurrence is mainly restricted to the subfamily Nepetoideae [31] and it is identified as one of the active components of several aromatic medicinal plants (e.g., *Salvia officinalis, Mentha* x *piperita, Lavandula officinalis, Ocimum basilicum, Origanum vulgare, Origanum majorana,* Thymus *vulgaris, Melissa officinalis, Rosmarinus officinalis*) [32]. For rosmarinic acid numerous and notable biological activities are confirmed in different *in vitro* and *in vivo* examinations. It is of pharmaceutical importance because of its non-specific complement activation and inhibition of the biosynthesis of leukotriens (leading to an anti-inflammatory effect), as well as its antimicrobial and especially antiviral activity [14, 33]. Additionally, it exhibits a very strong antioxidant effect; it is an inhibitor of acetyl and butyryl cholinesterase and neuroprotector that propose its use in the prevention and symptomatic treatment of Alzheimer's disease. However, it should be considered that bioavailability of rosmarinic acid in the brain is very unlikely. Also, in some test systems rosmarinic acid expresses anticarcinogenic activity [34, 35, 36].

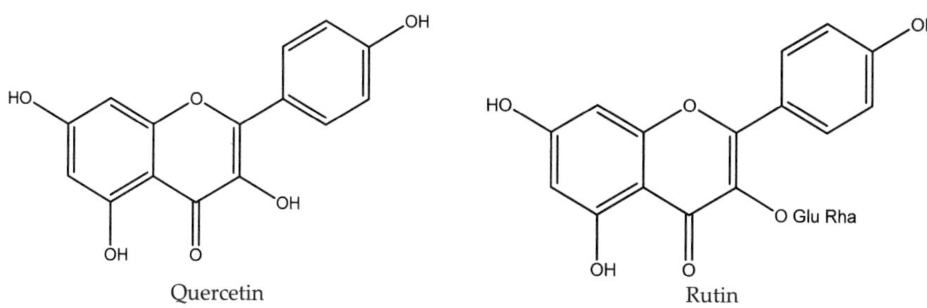

Figure 2. Chemical structures of flavonoids in investigated thyme extracts (Glu = glucose, Rha = rhamnose)

Extraction procedure	Identified compounds	References
Butanol-soluble fraction	Acetophenone glycosides (Androsin, Picein, glycosides of 4-hydroxyacetophenone derivatives)	[37]
Methanol, reflux, residue was extracted with distilled water at 100°C for 2 h	Acidic polysaccharide	[38]
Acetone using a Polytron homogenizer for 1 min	Caffeic acid, Luteolin, Rosmarinic acid, Hispidulin	[39]
CH_2Cl_2 soluble fraction	5,4`-Dihydroxy-6,7,8-trimethoxyflavone, 5,3`,4`-Trihydroxy-7-methoxyflavone, 5,4`-Dihydroxy-6,7,3`-trimethoxyflavone, 5,4`-Dihydroxy-6,7,8,3`-tetramethoxyflavone	[40]
Extracted at 20°C with 1L of EtOH-H_2O-HOAc (80:19:1) under N_2 for 5 days; further fractionation	Rosmarinic acid, 3`-*O*-(8``-Z-Caffeoyl) rosmarinic acid, Eriodictyol, Taxifolin, Luteoline-7-O-glucuronide	[41]

Extraction procedure	Identified compounds	References
Methanol; 1 day at room temperature	biphenyl compounds (e.g. 3,4,3`,4`-tetrahydroxy-5,5`-diisopropyl-2,2`-dimethylbiphenyl)	[42]
Deodorised aqueous extracts	Total phenolics (mg/g gallic acid equivalents)	[43]
Methanol extract	Monoterpene glucosides (p-Cymenol-9-O-β-glucoside, 2- and 5-O-β-glucosides of thymoquinol, angelicoidenol-O-β-glucoside); Arbutin	[44]
Ethanol/water (30:70, v/v) with the aid of sonication for 10 min	Rosmarinic acid, Caffeic acid	[45]
methanol extract	compounds related to hydroxyjasmone (e.g. 5-hydroxyjasmone-5-O-ß-glucoside) and simple phenol glucosides (3-Hydroxy-4-methoxyphenethyl-3-O-ß-glucoside, eugenol-O-ß-glucoside, syringin)	[46]
Methanol, 20 min, 60°C in a water bath with shaking	Luteolin-glucoside, Rosmarinic acid, Eriodictyol, Luteolin, Apigenin	[47]
Methanol, 6 h, Soxhlet apparatus	Oleanolic acid, Ursolic acid	[48]
aqueous extracts (boiling water), 30 min	Luteolin-7-O-glucuronide, Lithospermic acid, Rosmarinic acid, Caffeic acid	[49]
Aquous, aq. methanolic, methanolic (1:100 or 1:200); infusion, hot methanolic, usage of ultrasonic bath for 15 or 30 min	Arbutin, Hydroquinone, Naringenin, Naringenin-7-O-ß-glucoside, Narirutin, Eriodictyol, Eriodictyol-7-O-ß-glucoside, Eriocitrin, Hesperidin, Luteolin, Luteolin-7-O-ß-glucuronide, Luteolin-7-O-ß-rutinoside, Rosmarinic acid, Methyl rosmarinate, Caffeic acid	[50]
95% ethanol at 60°C for 2 h with stirring	Total phenolics (mg/g sinapic acid equivalents)	[51]
Liquid nitrogen powdered samples were extracted with acidified methanol	Caffeic acid, Rosmarinic acid	[52]

Table 3. Comparison of literature data on identified compounds in *Thymus vulgaris* leaves

Chlorogenic acid (5-O-caffeoylquinic acid) is a natural antioxidant that is produced in various plants as a response to pathogen microorganisms, different mechanical impairment, or excessive exposure to light (Figure 5) [53]. Due to these characteristics, chlorogenic acid found its use in pharmaceutical and food industries, as well as in cosmetology [54]. Gallic and ferulic acids are also proven antioxidant agents (Figure 3) [45].

Furthermore, many beneficial properties have been identified for flavonoids (e.g., quecetin and rutin as the most widely distributed in nature) (Figure 2), and one of the most popularly cited property is their antioxidant activity. Other actions that are proposed to contribute to their biological effects include chelating metal ions, stimulating phase II detoxifying enzyme activity, and inhibiting proliferation and inducing apoptosis. Also, for some of the flavonoids

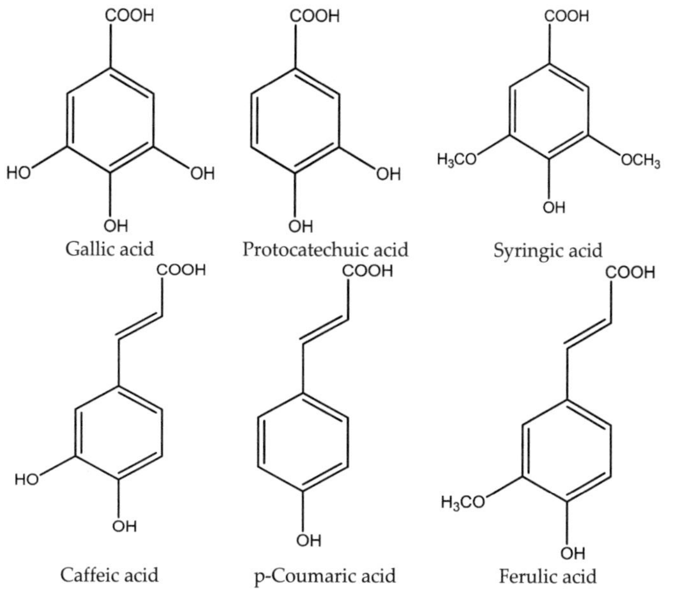

Figure 3. Chemical structures of hydroxybenzoic and hydroxycinnamic acids present in thyme extracts

where anti-inflammatory activity has been confirmed, they decrease the vascular cell adhesion and molecule expression, increase endothelial nitric oxide synthase activity, as well as inhibit platelet aggregation [55].

Specifically, it is determined that luteolin (3',4',5,7-tetrahydroxyflavone) exhibit notable antioxidant, antimicrobial, and anti-inflammatory activities [56]. Also, there is some evidence that apigenin and luteolin act as antimutagenic and anticarcinogenic agents (Figure 4) [57].

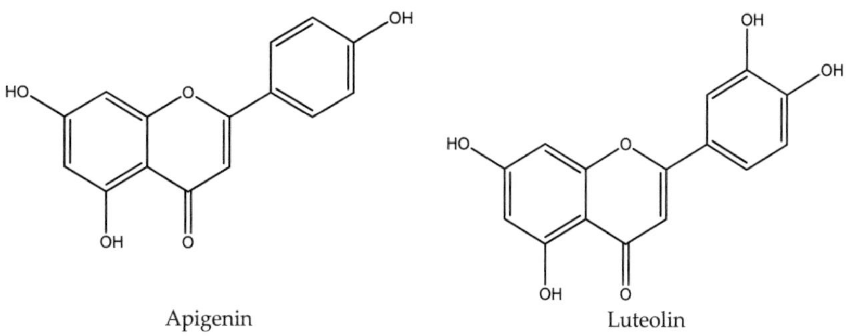

Figure 4. Chemical structures of dominant flavones in investigated thyme extracts

Since various plant extracts and isolated natural compounds are widely used and represent one of the major approaches in alternative and complementary medicine that are also accepted by conventional medicine, their quality, efficacy, and safety are of the utmost importance [58]. Safety issues are especially significant due to increasing body of evidence on side effects and interactions between herbal remedies or/and food or conventional drugs. These interactions sometimes can be very serious. They may lead to increased or lack of action of conventional drugs and caution must be taken in the application of plant extracts [59].

Nowadays, the biological potential of various plant waste materials is the focus of numerous studies. This trend includes not only the examination of aromatic plants [43, 60, 61, 62], but also different fruits and plant products such as wine, olives, beetroot, tomato, garlic, and pomegranate [63, 64, 65, 66]. These investigations also include their antimicrobial activity, considering the fact that waste material extracts represent the valuable source of different phenolic compounds. These studies are important, both in terms of economy and ecology, in order to elucidate the way to exploit post-distillation waste material of aromatic plants and other plant waste materials more efficiently.

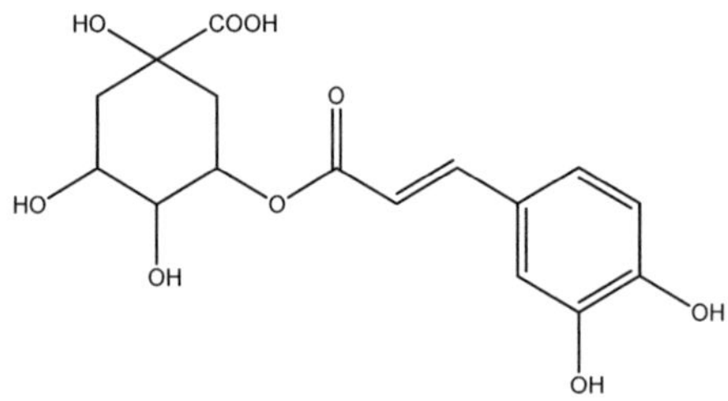

Chlorogenic acid

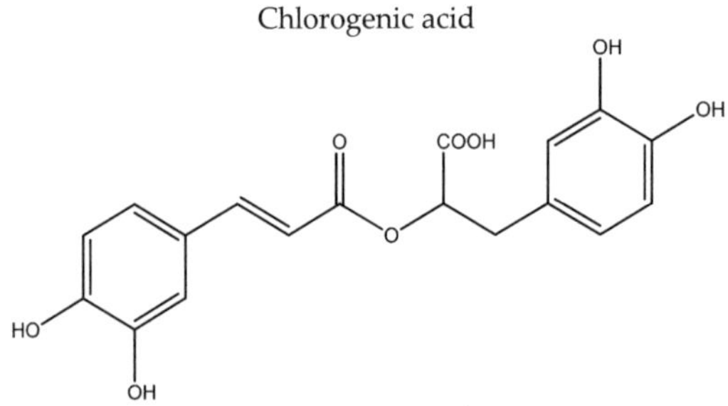

Rosmarinic acid

Figure 5. Chemical structures of dominant caffeic acid oligomers in thyme extracts

The aim of the present study was to determine the antibacterial potential of chemically well-characterised extracts obtained from waste material that remain after the preparation of the drug *Thymi folium* (stems) and the isolation of thyme essential oil (deodorised leaves and post-distillation decoction) on selected bacterial strains. Also, in order to determine the safety of the waste extracts, their cytotoxicity was investigated.

2. Methods

2.1. Plant material and extract preparation

In July 2013, aboveground parts of thyme (*Thymus vulgaris* L., Lamiaceae) were collected, just before flowering, in Padej, the Vojvodina province, Republic of Serbia. Voucher specimen of collected plants (no. ThV-15/10) [67] was confirmed and deposited at the Herbarium of the Laboratory of Pharmacognosy, Department of Pharmacy, Faculty of Medicine, University of Novi Sad. Leaves were separated from the previously air-dried stems and stored separately at a cool and dry place for extract preparation. Standard thyme leaves extract [15, 68] was prepared by maceration procedure in 45% ethanol (EtOH) as a solvent for 24 h (1:10 w/v, 10 g dried leaves) at room temperature (T1). Essential oil was isolated using hydrodistillation technique [69]. The waste material, remaining after isolation, was filtered and obtained decoction was used to prepare post-distillation extract (T2). Deodorised leaves were air dried and macerated with 45% (T3) and 75% (T4) EtOH for 24 h. Dried stems were grinded (sieve 0.75) and macerated with 45% EtOH for 24 h to obtain the extract T5.

After the maceration, extracts were collected, filtered, and evaporated to dryness under vacuum. The quantities of dry extracts were determined gravimetrically. Residues were dissolved in water to make 10% (w/v) stock solutions for further investigation. For the high-performance liquid chromatography (HPLC analysis), residues were dissolved in methanol, 1% formic acid mixture (50:50 v/v) to make 2% (w/v) stock solutions.

2.2. Chemical composition

2.2.1. Determination of total phenolic compounds and total flavonoid content

The amount of total phenolic compounds in investigated extracts was determined spectrophotometrically with Folin-Ciocalteu (FC) reagent [70]. The concentration of total phenolic compounds was expressed in mg of gallic acid equivalents (GAE) per g of dry extract (d.e.), using a standard curve of gallic acid (concentration range 0.08–0.24 mg/mL). Total flavonoid content was also determined spectrophotometrically using a method based on the formation of a flavonoid-aluminium complex with an absorptivity maximum at 430 nm [71]. Flavonoid content was expressed in mg of quercetin equivalents (QE) per g of dry extract, using a standard curve of quercetin (concentration range 10–100 μg/mL). All measurements were done in triplicate.

2.2.2. HPLC/DAD analysis

Investigated thyme leaves extracts are rich in a wide range of phenolic compounds [50]. Therefore, a method that allows simultaneous detection of various phenolics in a single run was developed. This decreases the time necessary for analysis and reduces the analysis costs [72]. HPLC analysis was performed using a liquid chromatograph (Agilent 1200 series), equipped with diode array detector (DAD) and Eclipse XDB-C18, 1.8 μm, 4.6×50 mm column, at a flow-rate of 1 mL/min. Solvent gradient was performed by varying the proportion of solvent A (methanol) to solvent B (1% formic acid inwater (v/v)) [73]. The total running time and post-running time were 45 and 10 min, respectively. The column temperature was 30ºC. The injected volume of samples and standards was 5 μL and it was done automatically using an autosampler. The spectra were acquired in the range of 210–400 nm and chromatograms plotted at 280, 330, and 350 nm with a bandwidth of 4 nm, and with reference wavelength/bandwidth of 500/100 nm. Quantification of selected phenolics: gallic acid, protocatechuic acid, caffeic acid, chlorogenic acid, syringic acid, *p*-coumaric acid, ferulic acid, rutin, rosmarinic acid, quercetin, and apigenin (Figure 6) were done using the calibration curve of standard compounds.

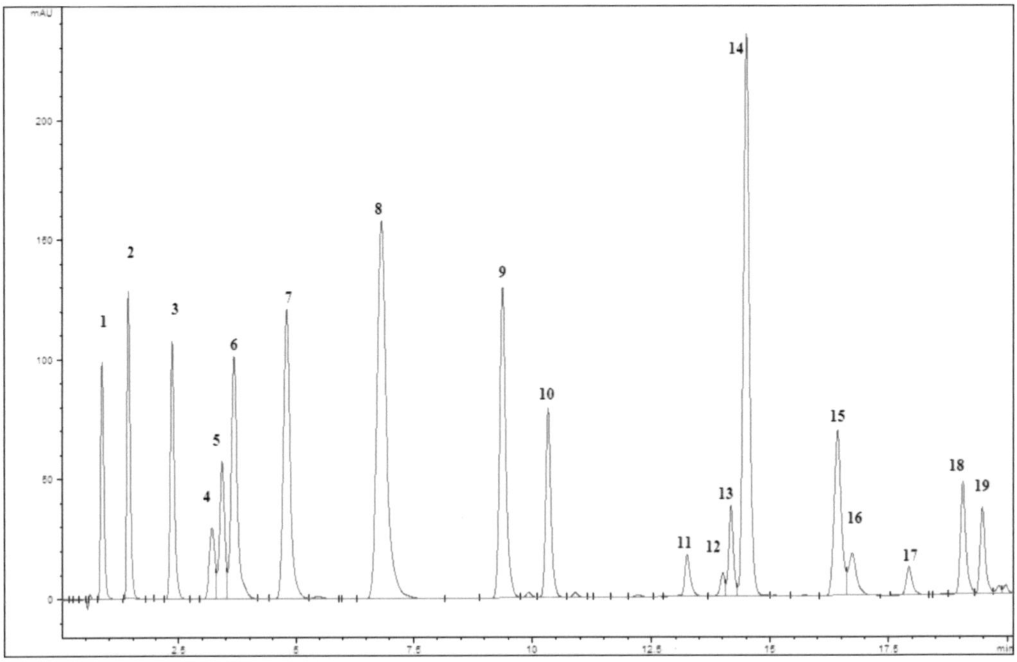

Figure 6. The chromatogram of the mixture of standards at 280nm used for chemical analysis of investigated thyme extracts. The order of elution of compounds was: 1-gallic acid, 2-protocatechuic acid, 3-*p*-hydroxybenzoic acid, 4-caffeic acid, 5-vanillic acid, 6-chlorogenic acid, 7-syringic acid, 8-*p*-coumaric acid, 9-ferulic acid, 10-sinapic acid, 11-rutin, 12-myricetin, 13-rosmarinic acid, 14-cinnamic acid, 15-quercetin, 16-naringenin, 17-luteolin 7-O-glucuronide, 18-kaemferol, 19-apigenin

2.3. Antibacterial testing

2.3.1. Bacterial strains and growth conditions

Selected bacterial strains, namely *Bacillus cereus* WSBC 10530 (clinical isolate), *Staphylococcus aureus* ATCC 25923 (clinical isolate), *Salmonella* Infantis ŽMJ 106 (poultry meat isolate), *Escherichia coli* O157:H7 ŽM 370 (clinical isolate), and *Campylobacter jejuni* NCTC 11168) were used for antibacterial testing. All bacterial strains were stored at –80°C. *B. cereus*, *S. aureus*, *S.* Infantis and *E. coli* were grown on Mueller-Hinton agar (MHA, Oxoid) at 37°C for 24 h. *C. jejuni* was grown on Columbia blood agar (Oxoid, Basingstoke, UK) at 42°C for 24 h under microaerobic conditions. For the antimicrobial activity assays, cultures were suspended in Mueller-Hinton broth (MHB, Oxoid) to 10^5–10^6 CFU/mL.

2.3.2. Broth microdilution method

Antimicrobial test systems should ideally be simple, reproducible, rapid, and inexpensive [74]. Several methods are currently available to determine antimicobial activity of different plant extracts or isolated pure compounds. Since they are not based on the same principle, the obtained results are influenced not only by the selected method, but also by the microorganism used, as well as by the extraction procedure (polar or non-polar extracts, essential oils, etc.) or the solubility of the tested compound [75]. In order to avoid overemphasizing the usefulness of various plant extracts or isolated compounds as antimicrobials, applied methods, both for extraction and antimicrobial testing, should be standardised to obtain comparable and reproducible results, prior to their *in vivo* application [76]. Broth macro- or microdilution methods for Minimum Inhibitory Concentration (MIC) determination are recommended by the Clinical and Laboratory Standards Institute (CLSI) [77]. In our study, micromethod, as it was less expensive and easier, was used to yield reproducible results. On the other hand, bacterial growth could be assessed visually, spectrophotometrically, or by using bioluminescence of fluorimetry measurements. However, all of the proposed methods have its shortcomings [78] and in this context colorimetric methods could represent an alternative approach, using tetrazolium salts as indicators. Bacteria convert them to coloured formazan derivatives that can be quantified, but difficulties may arise because of autofluorescence, salt reduction, and the antioxidant properties of plant products, especially for XTT (2,3-Bis-(2-Methoxy-4-nitro-5-sulfophenyl)-2H-tetrazolium-5-carboxanilide), TTC (2,3,5-triphenyl tetrazolium chloride), and resazurin. This makes them less convenient indicators for MIC assay. Therefore, INT (2-[4-iodophenyl]-3-[4-dinitrophenyl]-5-phenyltetrazolium chloride) was more suitable and was used in our survey. Change of colour occurs due to the reduction process as INT acts as an artificial terminal electron acceptor in respiration. Nevertheless, tetrazolium salts are not appropriate for microaerophilic campylobacters since they indicate the respiratory activity. Therefore, we used broth microdillution method with ATP measurement as rapid and accurate tools [74].

For the broth microdilution test, 50 μL of each bacterial suspension in suitable growth medium was added to the wells of a sterile 96-well microtitre plate already containing 50 μL of two-fold serially diluted standardised (T1) and post-distillation waste thyme extracts (T2, T3, T4, and T5) in proper growth medium. The final volume in each well was 100 μL. Control wells were prepared with culture medium, bacterial suspension only, plant extracts only, and ethanol in amounts corresponding to the highest quantity present. The contents of each well were mixed on a microplate shaker (Eppendorf, Hamburg, Germany) at 800 rpm for 1 min prior to incubation for 24 h in the cultivation conditions described above. The MIC was the lowest concentration where no viability was observed after 24 h on the basis of metabolic activity. To indicate respiratory activity, the presence of colour was determined after adding 10 μL/well of INT (Sigma) dissolved in water (INT 2 mg/mL) and incubated under appropriate cultivation conditions for 30 min in the dark [79]. To determine the ATP activity, the bioluminescence signal was measured by a Microplate Reader (Tecan, Mannedorf/Zurich, Switzerland) after adding 100 μL/well of BacTiter-Glo™ reagent (Promega, Madison, USA) after 5 min of the incubation in the dark [80]. Positive controls were wells with a bacterial suspension in an appropriate growth medium and a bacterial suspension in an appropriate growth medium with ethanol in amounts corresponding to the highest quantity present in the broth microdilution assay. Negative controls were wells with growth medium and plant extract. All measurements of MIC values were repeated in triplicate. Results are expressed in mg of total phenolics (TP).

2.4. Cytotoxicity studies

2.4.1. Cell culture

Human MRC-5 lung fibroblasts were grown in Minimum Essential Medium (MEM, Gibco, Invitrogen, Austria) supplemented with 2 mM of L-glutamine (Sigma, MO, USA), 10% of heat-inactivated fetal bovine serum (FBS, PAA laboratories, Austria), 100 units/mL of Penicillin (PAA laboratories), and 100 μg/mL of Streptomycin (PAA laboratories) (1% Pen/Strep). Cells were kept in a humidified 5% CO_2 atmosphere at 37°C and passaged at 90% confluence. Passages P26 and P27 were used for the assays.

2.4.2. XTT assay for the determination of cytotoxicity

An automated microculture tetrazolium assay (MTA) has long been used for the *in vitro* assessment of drug effects on cell growth. The use of the MTT (3-(4,5-dimethylthiazol-2-yl)-2,5-diphenyltetrazolium bromide) tetrazolium reagent requires dimethyl sulfoxide solubilization MTT-formazan generated by cellular reduction. This is not only laborious, but also may risk exposure of laboratory personnel to large quantities of potentially hazardous solutions in dimethyl sulfoxide (DMSO). Furthermore, frequent DMSO exposure also produces deleterious effects upon some laboratory equipment. Therefore, to allow the investigation of a simplified MTA and to address potential problems associated with solvent handling, a series of new tetrazolium salts have been developed which, upon metabolic reduction by viable cells, yield aqueous-soluble formazans [81]. One of the possible alternatives was found to be XTT (2,3-bis(2-methoxy-4-nitro-5-sulfophenyl)-S-[(phenylamino)carbonyl]-2H-tetrazolium hydroxide), which is metabolically reduced in viable cells to a water soluble formazan product. This allows reproducible estimates of drug sensitivity in a variety of human and other tumor cell lines. However, it is also applicable for the cytotoxicity studies of various natural products, such are plant extracts or isolated natural compounds.

Cell proliferation kit II (XTT) (Cat. No. 11 465 015 001) was obtained from Roche Diagnostics (Mannheim, Germany). Aliquots (100 μL) of $1x10^5$ cells/mL were seeded into 96 well plates (flat bottom) and grown for 24 h before the extracts were added. Afterwards, cells were incubated for 4 h or 24 h with investigated thyme extracts (20 μg/mL) before XTT solution was added. The XTT solution consisted of a XTT labeling reagent and an electron-coupling reagent and was always freshly prepared. XTT is a yellow tetrazolium salt and cleaved by metabolic active cells into an orange, water-soluble formazan dye. Since these color changes only occur in viable cells, it can be directly quantified using a scanning multiwell spectrophotometer [81]. Numbers of viable cells were determined with the following formula and expressed as percentage of control [82]:

Absorbance of treated cells/Absorbance of untreated cells x 100

Control cells represent vehicle-treated cells. Vehicle was 0.5% of DMSO (final concentration), which did not affect the cells as shown by control experiments.

2.4.3. Cytoprotection assay

Aliquots (100 μL) of 1x10^5 cells/mL were seeded into 96 well plates (flat bottom) and grown for 24 h before the extracts (20 μg/mL) were added for 4 h or 24 h. Afterwards, the medium with the extracts was removed and replaced by 100 μl of a H_2O_2 solution (50 μM, 100 μM, 200 μM or 500 μM) in MEM medium and further incubated for 2 h or 24 h. To finally determine the cell viability, XTT solution was added and analyzed as described above.

2.5. Statistical analysis

The data were reported as mean values ± standard deviation (SD) and processed using Microsoft Office Excel for Windows v. 2007.

3. Results

3.1. The amount of dry extract

The amounts of dry extracts obtained by maceration of thyme leaves (T1), deodorised thyme leaves (T3 and T4), and thyme stems (T5) and post-distillation extract remaining after the evaporation of thyme decoction (T2) are shown in Table 4. Generally, the amount of dry extract T1 is in accordance with previously published data, considering the fact that numerous factors could influence the extraction yield [47, 83]. When the thyme waste extracts were analyzed, the highest amount was obtained in T2 [43]. The difference in the extraction yield between T1 and T2 may be due to the mere extraction process since T2 is obtained after hydrodistillation of thyme leaves that favours extraction of polar substances, but also present carbohydrates genuine to the leaves or generated after hydrolysis of present glycosides. Deodorised leaves and stems yield a smaller amount of dry extracts when compared to T1.

3.2. Total phenolic compounds and flavonoid content

Spectrophotometric methods used are simple and reproducible for rough screening of total phenolic compounds and total flavonoids before detailed chemical analysis. The results are presented in Table 4. Total phenolic compounds in examined thyme leaves and stem extracts varied from 35.69 (T2) to 62.45 (T4) mg GAE/g d.e., while total flavonoids were in the 11.31 (T5)–52.89 (T3) mg QE/g d.e. range. Interestingly, deodorised leaves extracts (T3 and T4) have a relatively high content of total phenolic compounds and total flavonoids when compared to T1. The extract T2, for which the highest amount of dry extract was determined, is poor in total phenolic compounds and total flavonoids when compared to T1, but also to T3 and T4 [43, 51]. However, when absolute amounts (in plant material) are considered, T2 may also represent a valuable source of phenolic compounds and flavonoids. Stem extract (T5) have relatively high total phenolics, while are poor in total flavonoids.

Type of extract	% dry extract (g d.e./100 g of plant material)	Total phenolic compounds (mg GAE/g d.e.)	Total flavonoid content (μg QE/g d.e.)
T1	**9.31**±0.05	**49.71**±0.02	**33.88**±0.014
T2	**37.19**±0.1	**35.69**±0.019	**22.79**±0.005
T3	**3.45**±0.03	**58.23**±0.019	**52.89**±0.012
T4	**3.85**±0.04	**62.45**±0.006	**50.09**±0.006
T5	**5.39**±0.05	**45.95**±0.03	**11.31**±0.005

Table 4. The amount of dry extract, total phenolic compounds, and total flavonoid content

3.3. HPLC analysis

The qualitative-quantitative data from the chromatographic analyses are presented in Table 5, with representative chromatograms for T1 and T3 (Figure 7). The following components: gallic, protocatechuic, caffeic, chlorogenic, syringic, *p*-coumaric, ferulic, and rosmarinic acid, as well as rutin, quercetin, luteolin 7-O-glucuronide andapigenin were identified and quantified within the investigated samples.

Type of extract c (mg/g d.e.)	T1	T2	T3	T4	T5
Gallic acid	2.46	2.58	1.76	0.77	4.99
Protocatechuic acid	0.23	0.22	0.27	0.37	0.22
Caffeic acid	0.35	0.23	0.13	0.33	0.53
Chlorogenic acid	2.06	2.02	3.77	4.75	7.75
Syringic acid	0.23	0.42	0.3	0.36	0.25
p-Coumaric acid	0.06	0.04	0.05	0.06	0.16
Ferulic acid	1.05	0.89	1.56	1.9	5.77
Rutin	0.4	0.12	2.4	3.68	0.32
Rosmarinic acid	**62.22**	**60.49**	**86.01**	**105.08**	**52.36**
Quercetin	0.35	0.04	2.2	3.98	0.36
Luteolin 7-O-glucuronide	**42.20**	**34.44**	**81.24**	**87.11**	**11.01**
Apigenin	1.81	0.79	3.36	4.45	0.27

Table 5. Results of HPLC-DAD analysis of thyme leaves and post-distillation waste extracts

Regarding the hydroxybenzoic, hydroxycinnamic acids, and caffeic acid oligomers, rosmarinic acid was identified as the major component in all the investigated thyme extracts and was present within the range of 52.36 (T5) to 105.08 (T4) mg/g d.e, which is similar to the previously published data for officially prepared thyme extracts (T1) [50]. Also, gallic, ferulic, and chlorogenic acids were present in considerable amounts. In general, 75% EtOH extract of the deodorised leaves (T4) abundant in rosmarinic, chlorogenic, and ferulic acid, whilst 45% EtOH contained higher amounts of gallic acid. In the flavonoid fraction, luteolin 7-O-glucuronide was the dominant and the second major identified component in all investigated extracts (from 11.01 (T5) to 87.11 (T4) mg/g d.e.). Similarly to the total phenolic content, the highest amounts of almost all quantified components, especially the dominant ones were determined in deodorised leaves extracts (T3 and T4). Also, although the stem is confirmed to be relatively poor in phenolic compounds, chlorogenic and ferulic acids are present in considerable amounts.

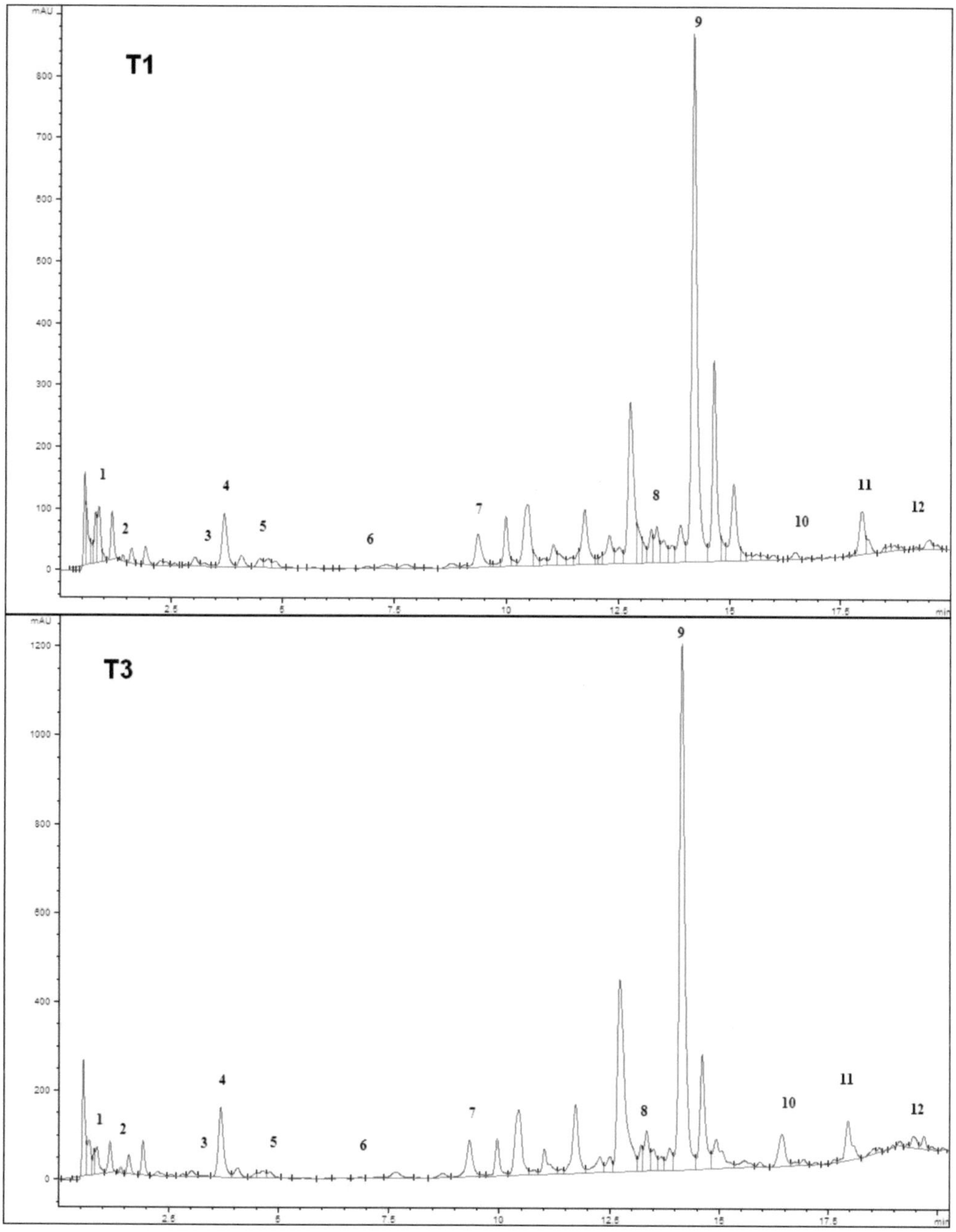

Figure 7. Chromatograms of examined thyme leaves extracts (T1 and T3) at 280 nm: 1-gallic acid, 2-protocatechuic acid, 3-caffeic acid, 4- chlorogenic acid, 5-syringic acid, 6-*p*-coumaric acid, 7- ferulic acid, 8-rutin, 9-rosmarinic acid, 10-quecetin, 11-luteolin 7-O-glucuronide, 12-apigenin

3.4. Antibacterial testing

Numerous studies have confirmed the use of herbs and spices as anti-infective agents [84]. Among them, different essential oils and phenolic compounds, or plant extracts rich in phenolic compounds stand out for their antibacterial activity [85, 86]. This is particularly important, given that phenolic compounds possess a strong antioxidant potential. This joint action is significant for their usage in pharmaceutical and food industries, but also in all other fields where it is important to prevent both oxidation and contamination of certain products [87].

All investigated post-distillation thyme waste extracts exhibited relatively strong antimicrobial potential, against all tested bacterial strains, especially deodorised leaves extracts (T3 and T4) (Table 6) [88]. Also, thyme stem extract (T5) expressed notable antibacterial action. What is more important, by comparing these results with the data obtained for butylhydroxytoluene (BHT), often used as a synthetic additive, antibacterial potential of thyme post-distillation waste material extracts becomes even more evident. Also, interestingly, all investigated thyme extracts showed lower minimal inhibitory concentration on all investigated bacterial strains when compared to isolated rosmarinic acid. This may indicate that phenolic compounds possess a synergistic antibacterial effect, which is important in terms of emerging occurrence of resistance.

	Staphylococcus aureus MIC (mg TP/mL)	*Salmonella liverpool* MIC (mg TP/mL)	*Escherichia coli* MIC (mg TP/mL)	*Bacillus cereus* MIC (mg TP/mL)
T1	0.09	0.28	0.14	0.14
T2	0.14	0.39	0.56	1.55
T3	**0.04**	**0.12**	**0.12**	**0.03**
T4	**0.06**	**0.12**	**0.12**	**0.03**
T5	0.09	0.13	0.19	0.06
BHT (mg/mL)	0.55	0.55	0.55	0.28
Rosmarinic acid*	5	2.5	2.5	5

* reference [74]

Table 6. Minimal inhibitory concentrations of investigated thyme extracts on selected bacterial strains

Despite many recent technological advances in the food industry, which have contributed to increased safety in the food supply chain, we are still facing high incidence of foodborne illnesses. In 2011 alone, there were 69,553 human cases originating from foodborne zoonotic outbreaks in the EU [89]. Ninety-three of them were fatal. In the same year, *Campylobacter*, the most prevalent foodborne zoonotic agent, which is especially a problem in the production and processing of meat, caused 220 of the 209 registered, mostly sporadic human illnesses. It is assumed that the real burden is even much higher [4].

Two selected extracts, T3 prepared from deodorised leaves and T1 as an officially prepared one, were tested against *Campylobacter jejuni*. Both T1 and T3 expressed relatively strong antibacterial potential. The activity of deodorised extract T3 in gram negative *C. jejuni* was comparable to that in gram positive *S. aureus* and *B. cereus*. On the other hand, standard thyme extract T1 expressed substantially stronger activity in *C. jejuni* compared to all other tested species, suggesting that the phenolic compounds present in standard extract T1 may contribute more to the antimicrobial activity in *C. jejuni* than in other species. Furthermore, obtained MIC values of extracts were lower in comparison with rosmarinic acid, indicating the importance of synergistic effects of different compounds present in investigated extracts that can contribute to the antimicrobial activity through different mechanisms. They can interfere with bacterial membrane and thereby increase the cell leakage or act indirectly antimicrobial by facilitating the influx of antimicrobial phenolic compounds [21]. In this, as well as the economical aspect, the use of plant extracts might be more sensible than the use of pure compounds. However, obtained MIC values were much higher than those of selected antibiotics (Table 7).

	Campylobacter jejuni	References
T1	0.05	[88]
T3	0.06	[88]
Rosmarinic acid	1.25	[74]
Ciprofloxacin	0.25	[4]
Erythromycin	0.25	[4]

Table 7. Minimal inhibitory concentrations of selected thyme extracts (mg TP/mL), rosmarinic acid (mg/mL) and selected antibiotics (μg/mL) on *Camphylobacter jejuni*

3.5. Cytotoxicity studies

Cancer is a leading cause of death worldwide and sustained focus is on the discovery and development of newer and better-tolerated anti-cancer drugs, especially from plants. About 50% of all anti-cancer drugs approved internationally are either natural products or natural product mimics. They were developed on the basis of the knowledge obtained from small or macromolecules existing in nature [90].

The major challenges associated with currently available anti-cancer agents include selectivity, toxicity, resistance, and development of a secondary malignancy. These drawbacks have motivated the search for newer, more efficacious, and better tolerated anti-tumor drugs, with natural products, especially plants, offering an inexhaustible reservoir for new drug discovery and development. Also, molecular targeted agents are currently being studied in all treatment settings including that of chemoprevention, which is defined as the use of natural or synthetic nonessential dietary agents to interrupt the process of carcinogenesis and to prevent or delay tumor growth [91].

In vitro cytotoxicity studies are the first step in selecting from the vast number of still unexamined plant extracts or isolated compounds. Also, these studies can provide a valuable insight in the safety of different natural products. This is especially important for waste plant material, in our case for pos-tdistillation waste material of thyme leaves, if their possible future application in pharmaceutical or food industry should be considered.

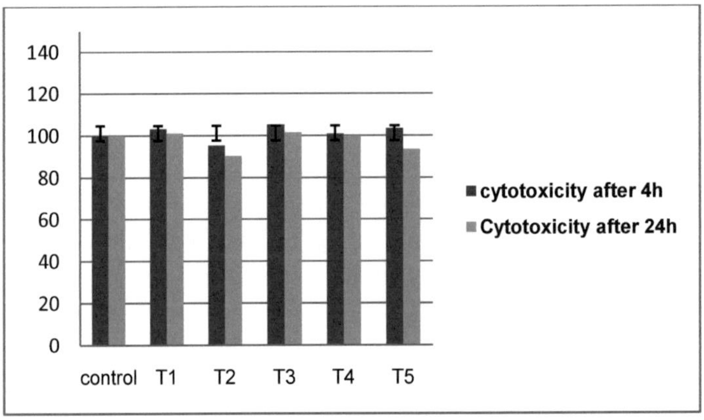

Figure 8. Metabolically active cells (% of control) in XTT assay after post-distillation thyme extracts application

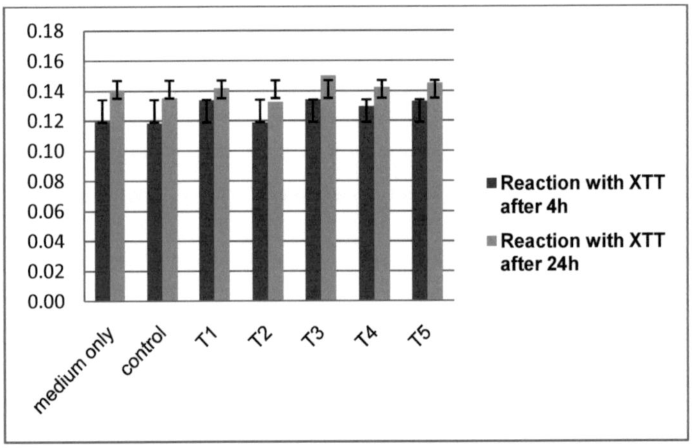

Figure 9. Absorbance values (490–650 nm) of extracts mixed with XTT solution in culture medium

The effects of investigated post-distillation thyme waste extracts against human MRC-5 lung fibroblasts are presented in Figures 8–15. Cytotoxicity of the extracts, a possible reaction with the XTT solvent and a potential cytoprotective activity were evaluated. As shown in Figure 8, none of the investigated extracts at concentrations of 20 μg/ml exhibited cytotoxicity after 4 h or 24 h of incubation. To exclude a direct reaction of the extracts with the XTT solvent and, therefore, false-negative results, extracts and XTT solution were mixed in culture medium and incubated for 4 h or 24 h. There were no significant differences in the absorbance values of medium and XTT alone compared to DMSO (control) or extracts (20 μg/ml) in medium (Figure 9) that reveals that the extracts did not interact with the XTT solution.

Finally, a potential cytoprotective effect of the extracts was investigated. Cells were incubated with the extracts for 4 h or 24 h and cytoprotection was evaluated by adding different concentrations of H_2O_2, which is a well-known cell damaging agent causing oxidative stress.

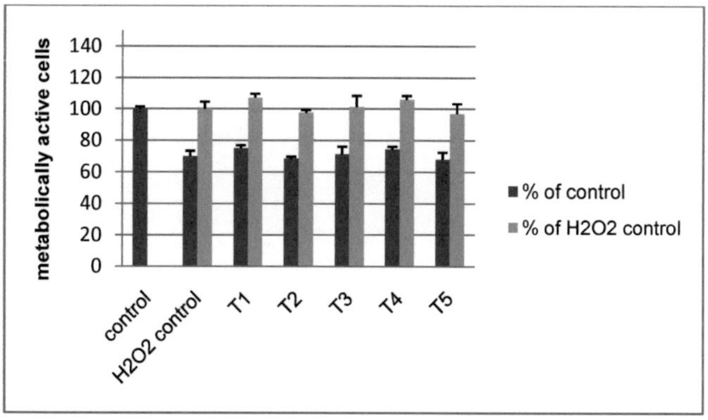

Figure 10. Cells incubated with the extracts for 24 h, medium replaced by 50 μM H_2O_2 and further incubated for 4 h (XTT added after 2h and read out after 2h)

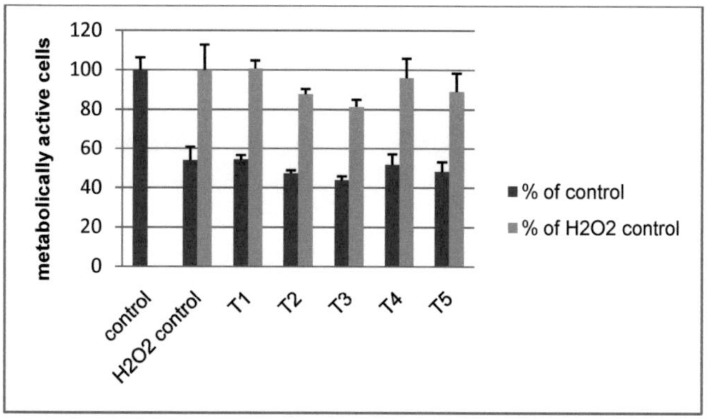

Figure 11. Cells incubated with the extracts for 24 h, medium replaced by 100 μM H_2O_2 and further incubated for 4h (XTT added after 2 h and read out after 2 h)

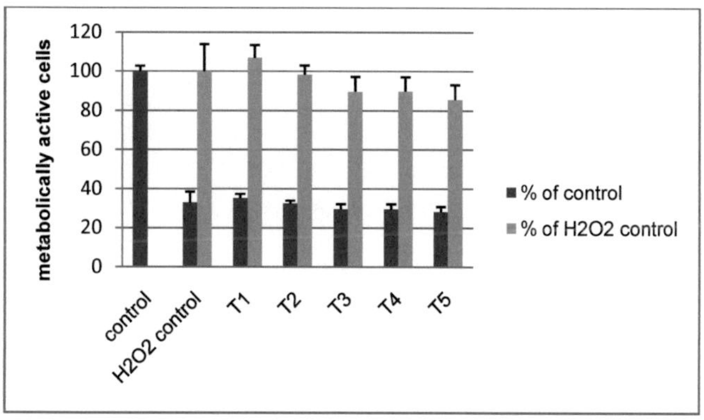

Figure 12. Cells incubated with the extracts for 24 h, medium replaced by 200 μM H_2O_2 and further incubated for 4h (XTT added after 2 h and read out after 2 h)

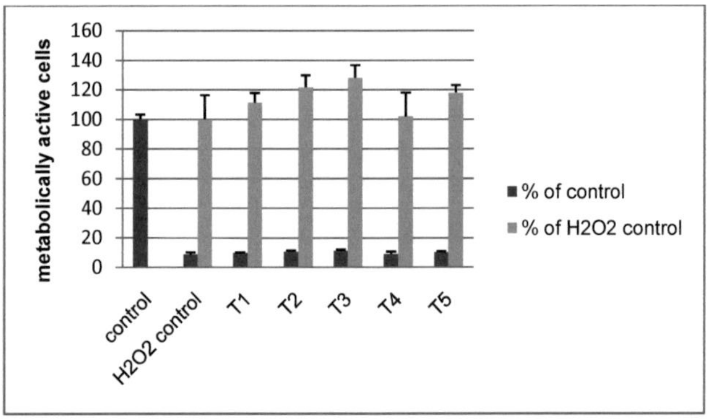

Figure 13. Cells incubated with the extracts for 24 h, medium replaced by 500 μM H_2O_2 and further incubated for 4 h (XTT added after 2 h and read out after 2 h)

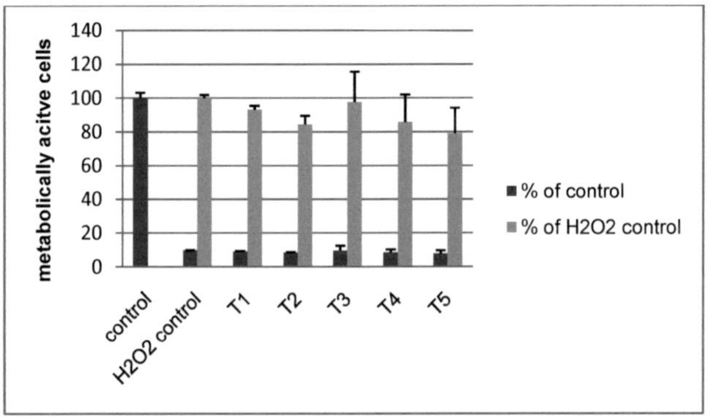

Figure 14. Cells incubated with the extracts for 4 h, medium replaced by 500 μM H_2O_2 and further incubated for 4 h (XTT added after 2 h and read out after 2 h)

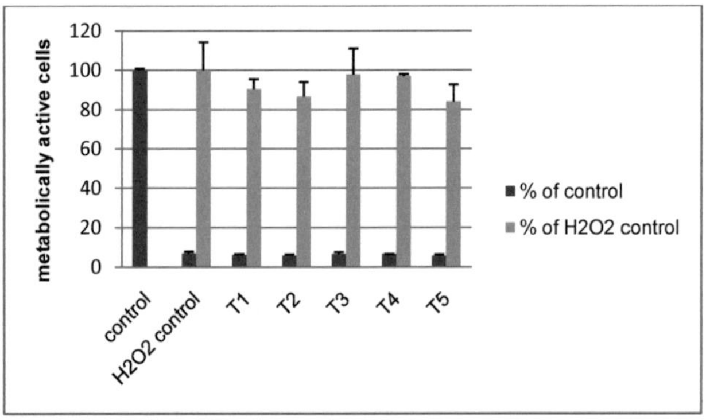

Figure 15. Cells incubated with the extracts for 4 h, medium replaced by 500 μM H_2O_2 and further incubated for 24 h (XTT added after 24 h and read out after 2 h)

The effects were compared to vehicle-treated (DMSO) cells (control) and to H_2O_2 treated cells (H_2O_2 control). As shown in Figures 10–15, none of the investigated extracts exhibited notable cytoprotective activity.

http://dx.doi.org/10.5772/60869

4. Further research

Results of microbiological tests indicate the possibility to use thyme postdistillation waste extracts primarily in the food or pharmaceutical industry as natural additives, regarding the relatively strong antibacterial activity on investigated bacterial strains.

Also, examined extracts represent a valuable source of phenolcarboxylic acids and flavonoids, which have numerous biological effects. Therefore thyme post-distillation waste material could be used for the isolation of rosmarinic acid and luteolin 7-O-glucuronide, as dominant compounds.

However, only limited data are presently available on the antimicrobial activity of plant extract in food systems and this indicates continuation of our study and the need for further work. Additionally, there is growing evidence on synergistic action of different plant products (extracts, essential oils, isolated compounds) with each other or with conventional antibiotics used in human and veterinary medicine [92]. Besides, it would be very interesting to collect more data on the efficiency of both thyme essential oil and investigated thyme extracts as a dietary supplementation in animal feed on protective or prebiotic effects on the gut microflora. Also, it is important to test their influence on antioxidant and antimicrobial stability and shelf life of meat and meat products [93, 94, 95].

Furthermore, the results of our study recorded neither cytotoxicity, nor cytoprotection of examined extracts. Yet, detailed in vivo toxicology analyses are required in order to confirm the safety of usage of thyme postdistillation waste material.

Acknowledgements

The authors are thankful to the research agencies of Slovenia, Serbia, and Austria for financing the bilateral projects BI-034-SLO-SR-2010/2011 and WTZ SI 03/2011 and to the The Provincial Secretariat for Science and Technological Development of Vojvodina (grant number: 114-451-2056/2011-01).

Author details

Neda Gavarić[1], Jasna Kovač[2], Nadine Kretschmer[3], Nebojša Kladar[1], Sonja Smole Možina[2], Franz Bucar[3], Rudolf Bauer[3] and Biljana Božin[1*]

*Address all correspondence to: bbozin2003@gmail.com

1 Department of Pharmacy, Faculty of Medicine, University of Novi Sad, Novi Sad, Serbia

2 Department of Food Science and Technology, Biotechnical Faculty, University of Ljubljana, Ljubljana, Slovenia

3 Institute of Pharmaceutical Sciences, Department of Pharmacognosy, University of Graz, Graz, Austria

References

[1] Rios JL, Recio MC. Medicinal plants and antimicrobial activity. Journal of Ethnopharmacology 2005;100 80–84.

[2] Reverter M,Bontemps N, Lecchini D, Banaigs B, Sasal P. Use of plant extracts in fish aquaculture as an alternative to chemotherapy: Current status and future perspectives. Aquaculture 2014;433 50–61.

[3] Palaniappan K, Holley RA. Use of natural antimicrobials to increase antibiotic susceptibility of drug resistant bacteria. International Journal of Food Microbiology 2010;140 164–168.

[4] Kovač J, Gavarić N, Bucar F, Smole Možina S. Antimicrobial and resistance modulatory activity of *Alpinia katsumadai* seed phenolic extract, essential oil and post-distillation extract. Food Technology and Biotechnology, 2014;52(2) 248–254.

[5] Singer RS, Williams-Nguyen J. Human health impacts of antibiotic use in agriculture: A push for improved causal inference. Current Opinions in Microbiology 2014;19 1–8.

[6] Machado TB, Pinto AV, Pinto MC, Leal IC, Silva MG, Amaral AC, Kuster RM, Netto-dos Santos KR. *In vitro* activity of Brazilian medicinal plants, naturally occurring naphthoquinones and their analogues, against methicilin-resistant *Staphylococcus aureus*. International Journal of Antimicrobial Agents 2003;21 279–284.

[7] Voravuthikunchai S, Lortheeranuwat A, Jeeju W, Sririrak T, Phongpaichit S, Supawita T. Effective medicinal plants against enterohaemorrhagic *Escherichia coli* O157:H7. Journal of Ethnopharmacology 2004;94 49–54.

[8] Fukai T, Oku Y, Hano Y, Terada S. Antimicrobial activites of hydrophilic 2-arylbenzofurans and an isoflavone against vancomycin-resistant enterococci and methicilin-resistant *Staphylococcus aureus*. Planta Medica 2004;70 685–687.

[9] Rani P, Khullar N. Antimicrobial evaluation of some medicinal plants for their anti-enteris potential against multi-drug resistant *Salmonella typhi*. Phytotherapy Research 2004;18 670–673.

[10] Shibata H, Kondo K, Katsuyama R, Kawazoe K, Sato Y, Murakami K, Takaishi Y, Arakaki N, Higuti T. Alkyl gallates, intensifiers of beta-lactam susceptibility in methicilin-resistant *Staphylococcus aureus*. Antimicrobial Agents and Chemotherapy 2005;49 549–555.

[11] Garcia-Garcia R, Lopez-Malo A, Palou E. Bactericidal action of binary and ternary mixtures of carvacrol, thymol, and eugenol against *Listeria innocua*. Journal of Food Science 2011;76 95–100.

[12] Gavaric N, Smole Možina S, Kladar N, Božin B. Chemical profile, antioxidant and antibacterial activity of thyme and oregano essential oils, thymol and carvacrol and

their possible synergism. Journal of Essential Oil Bearing Plants 2015;doi: 10.1080/0972060X.2014.971069.

[13] Mimica-Dukic N, Bozin N. Essential oils from Lamiaceae species as promising antioxidant and antimicrobial agents. Natural Product Communications 2007;2(4) 445–452.

[14] Heinrich M, Barnes J, Gibbons S, Williamson EM. Fundamentals of Pharmacognosy and Phytotherapy. Edinburgh, London, New York, Oxford, Philadelphia, St Louis, Sydney, Toronto: Churchill Livingstone; 2004.

[15] *European Pharmacopoea*. 6th edition. Strasbourgh: European Directorate for the Quality of Medicines & Health Care, Council of Europe; 2007.

[16] Božin B, Mimica-Dukić N, Simin N, Anačkov G. Characterization of the volatile composition of essential oils of some Lamiaceae spices and the antimicrobial and antioxidant activities of the entire oils. Journal of Agricultural and Food Chemistry 2006;54 1822–1828.

[17] Pirbalouti AG, Hashemi M, Ghahfarokhi FT. Essential oil and chemical compositions of wild and cultivated *Thymus daenensis* Celak and *Thymus vulgaris* L. Industrial Crops and Products 2013;48 43–48.

[18] Bozin B, Mimica-Dukic N, Anackov G, Zlatkovic B, Igic R. Variability of Content and Composition of *Mentha aquatica* L. (Lamiaceae) Essential Oil in Different Phenophases. Journal of Essential Oil Bearing Plants 2006a;9(3) 223–229.

[19] Bozin B, Mimica-Dukic N, Bogavac M, Suvajdzic L, Simin N, Samojlik I, Couladis M. Chemical composition, antioxidant and antibacterial properties of Achillea collina Becker ex Heimerl s.l. and A. pannonica Scheele essential oils. Molecules 2008;13(9) 2058–2068.

[20] Nabavi SM, Marchese A, Izadi M, Curti V, Daglia M, Nabavi SF. Plants belonging to the genus Thymus as antibacterial agents: From farm to pharmacy. Food Chemistry 2015;173 339-347.

[21] Burt S. Essential oils: Their antibacterial properties and potential applications in foods-a review. International Journal of Food Microbiology 2008;94 223–253.

[22] Tepe B, Deferera D, Sokmen M, Polissiou M, Sokmen A. *In vitro* antimicrobial and antioxidant activities of the essential oils and various extracts of *Thymus eigii* M. Zohary et P. H. Davis. Journal of Agricultural and Food Chemistry 2004;52 1132–1137.

[23] Rivas L, McDonnell MJ, Burgess CM, O'Brien M, Navarro-Villa A, Fanning S, Duffy G. Inhibition of verocytotoxigenic Escherichia coli in model broth and rumen systems by carvacrol and thymol. International Journal of Food Microbiology 2010;139 70–8.

[24] FDA. US Food and Drug Administration. www.cfsan.fda.gov/~dms/eafus.html. 2010.

[25] Booth N, Kruger C, Wallace Hayes A, Clemens R. An innovative approach to the safety evaluation of natural products: Cranberry leaf aqueous extracts as a case study. Food and Chemical Toxicology 2012;50 3150–3165.

[26] Jeršek B, Anđić M, Markov K, Lakić N, Božin B, Smole Možina S. Antifungal effect of essential oils on *Aspergillus westerdijkiae, A. ochraceus, A. flavus* and *Penicillium nordicum*. 6th Central European Congress on Food, Novi Sad, Serbia: May 2012.

[27] Božin B, Lakić N, Srđenović Čonić B, Kladar N, Orčić D, Mimica-Dukić N. Antioxidant and antimicrobial properties of a new chemotype of woodland sage (*Salvia nemorosa* L. subsp. *nemorosa*, Lamiaceae) essential oil. Biologica Serbica 2012;1–2(34) 51–60.

[28] Calo JR, Crandall PG, O'Bryan CA, Ricke SC, Essential oils as antimicrobials in food systems-a review. Food Control 2015;doi:10.1016/j.foodcont.2014.12.040.

[29] Bozin B, Mimica-Dukic N, Samojlik I, Jovin E. Antimicrobial and antioxidant properties of Rosemary and Sage (Rosmarinus officinalis L. and Salvia officinalis L., Lamiaceae) essential oils. Journal of Agricultural and Food Chemistry 2007;55(19) 7879–7885.

[30] Samojlik I, Lakić N, Mimica-Dukić N, Đaković-Švajcer K, Božin B. Antioxidant and Hepatoprotective Potential of Essential Oils of Coriander (*Coriandrum sativum* L.) and Caraway (*Carum carvi* L.) (Apiaceae). Journal of Agricultural and Food Chemistry 2010;58 8848–8853.

[31] Takhtajan A. Flowering Plants. Berlin: Springer Verlag; 2009.

[32] Petersen M, Abdullah Y, Benner J, Eberle D, Gehlen K, Hücherig S, Janiak V, Kim KH, Sander M, Weitzel C, Wolters S. Evolution of rosmarinic acid biosynthesis. Phytochemistry. 2009,70(15–16) 1663–1679.

[33] Nolkemper S, Reichling J, Stintzing FC, Carle R, Schnitzler P. Antiviral effect of aqueous extracts from species of the Lamiaceae family against Herpes simplex virus type 1 and type 2 in vitro. Planta Medica 2006;72(15) 1378–1382.

[34] Akhondzadeh, S. Abbasi, SH. Herbal medicine in treatment of Alzheimer's disease. American Journal of Alzheimer's Disease and Other Dementias 2006;21 113–118.

[35] Lee HJ, Cho H, Park E, Kim S, Lee S, Kim C, Kim DK, Kim S, Chun HS. Rosmarinic acid protects human dopaminergic neuronal cells against hydrogen peroxide-induced apoptosis. Toxicology 2008;250 109–115.

[36] Dastmalchi K, Ollilainen V, Lackman P, Boije af Gennäs G, Damien Dorman, HJ, Järvinen P, Yli-Kauhaluoma J, Hiltunen R. Acetylcholinesterase inhibitory guided fractionation of *Melissa officinalis* L. Bioorganic & Medicinal Chemistry 2009;17 867–871.

[37] Wang H, Kikuzaki H, Lin CC, Kahyaoglu A, Huang MT, Nakatani N. Acetophenone glycosides from thyme (*Thymus vulagris* L.). Journal of Agricultural and Food Chemistry 1999;47 1911–1914.

[38] Chun H, Jun WJ, Shin DH, Hong BS, Cho HY, Yang HC. Purification and characterization of anti-complementary polysaccharide from leaves of *Thymus vulgaris* L. Chemical and Pharmaceutical Bulletin 2001;49 762–764.

[39] Zheng W, Wang SY. Antioxidant activity and phenolic compounds in selected herbs. Journal of Agricultural and Food Chemistry 2001;49(11) 5165–5170.

[40] Miura K, Kikuzaki H, Nakatani N. Antioxidant activity of chemical components from sage (*Salvia officinali*L.) and thyme (*Thymus vulgaris* L.) measured by the oil stability index method. Journal of Agricultural and Food Chemistry 2002;50 1845–1851.

[41] Depkevicius A, Van Beek TA, Lelyveld GP, Van Veldhuizen A, De Groot A, Linssen JPH, Venskutonis R. Isolation and structure elucidation of radical scavengers from *Thymus vulgaris* leaves. Journal of Natural Products 2002;65 892–896.

[42] Okazaki K, Kawazoe K, Takaishi Y. Human platelet aggregation inhibitors from thyme (*Thymus vulgaris* L.). Phytotherapy Research 2002;16 398–399.

[43] Dorman HJD, Peltoketo A, Hiltunen R, Tikkanen MJ. Characterisation of the antioxidant properties of de-odourised aqueous extracts from selected Lamiaceae herbs. Food Chemistry 2003;83 255–262.

[44] Tagashira M, Ohtake Y. New monoterpene glucosides from aerial parts of thyme (*Thymus vulgaris* L.). Planta Medica 1998;64 555–558.

[45] Wang H, Provan GJ, Halliwell K. Determination of rosmarinic acid and caffeic acid in aromatic herbs by HPLC. Food Chemistry 2004;87 307–311.

[46] Kitajima J, Ishikawa T, Urabe A. A new hydroxyjasmone glucoside and its related compounds from the leaf of thyme. Chemical and Pharmaceutical Bulletin 2004;52 1013–1014.

[47] Kosar M, Dorman HJD, Hiltunen R. Effect of acid treatment on the phytochemical and antioxidant characteristics of extracts from selected Lamiaceae species. Food Chemistry 2005;91 522–533.

[48] Janicsak G, Mathe I, Miklossay-Vari V, Blunden G. Comparative studies of the rosmarinic and caffeic acid contents of Lamiaceae species. Biochemical Systematics and Ecology 1999;27 733–738.

[49] Fecka I, Raj D, Krauze-Baranowska M. Quantitative determination of four water-soluble compounds in herbal drugs from Lamiaceae using different chromatographic techniques. Chromatographia 2007;66 87–93.

[50] Fecka I, Turek S. Determination of polyphenolic compounds in commercial herbal drugs and spices from Lamiaceae: Thyme, wild thyme and sweet marjoram by chromatographic techniques. Food Chemistry 2008;108 1039–1053.

[51] Amarowicz R, Zegarska Z, Rafalowski R, Pegg RB, Karamac M, Kosinska A. Antioxidant activity and free radical-scavenging capacity of ethanolic extracts of thyme, oregano and marjoram. European Journal of Lipid Science and Technology 2009;111 1111–1117.

[52] Lee J. Caffeic acid derivatives in dried Lamiaceae and *Echinacea purpurea* products. Journal of Functional Foods 2010;2 158–162.

[53] Farah A, Danangelo CM. Phenolic compounds in coffee. Brazilian Journal of Plant Physiology 2006;18 23–36.

[54] Marques V, Farah A. Chlorogenic acids and related compounds in medicinal plants and infusions. Food Chemistry 2009;113 1370–376.

[55] Dewick P. Medicinal natural Products. John Wiley & Sons; 2002.

[56] Kobayashi R, Itou T, Hanaya K, Shoji M, Hada N, Sugai T.Chemo-enzymatic transformation of naturally abundant naringin to luteolin, a flavonoid with various biological effects. Journal of Molecular Catalysis B: Enzymatic 2013;92 14–18.

[57] Lin J, Chen Y, Lee Y, Rolis Hou C, Chen F, Yang D. Antioxidant, anti-proliferative and cyclooxygenase-2 inhibitory activities of ethenolic extracts from lemon balm (*Melissa officinalis* L.) leaves. LWT-Food Science and Technology 2012;49 1–7.

[58] Samojlik I, Mijatović V, Gavarić N, Krstin S, Božin B. Consumers' attitude towards the use and safety of herbal medicines and herbal dietary supplements in Serbia. International Journal of Clinical Pharmacy 2013;35 835-840.

[59] Williamson E, Driver S, Baxter K, editors. Stockley's herbal medicines interactions. London: Pharmaceutical Press; 2009.

[60] Božin B, Lakić N, Mišan A, Smole Možina S. Phenolic profile, antioxidant and antimicrobial activity of oregano (*Origanum vulgare* L., Lamiaceae) postdistillation waste extracts, 6th Central European Congress on Food, Novi Sad, Serbia: May 2012.

[61] Peev G, Penchev P, Peshev D, Angelov G. Solvent extraction of rosmarinic acid from lemon balm and concentration of extracts by nanofiltration: Effect of plant pre-treatment by supercritical carbon dioxide. Chemical Engineering Research and Design 2011;89 2236–2243.

[62] Dzamic A, Sokovic M, Novakovic M, Jadranin M, Ristic M, Tesevic V, Marin P. Composition, antifungal and antioxidant properties of *Hyssopus officinalis* L. subsp. *pilifer* (Pant.) Murb.Essential oil and deodorized extracts. Industrial Crops and Products 2013;51 401–407.

[63] Cioffi G, Pesca MS, De Caprariis P, Braca A, Severino L, De Tommasi N. Phenolic compounds in olive oil and olive pomace from Cilento (Campenia, Italy) and their antioxidant activity. Food Chemistry 2010;121(1) 105–111.

[64] Sagdic O, Ozturk I, Ozkan G, Yetim H, Ekici L, Yilmaz MT. RP-HPLC-DAD analysis of phenolic compounds in pomace extracts from five grape cultivars: Evaluation of their antioxidant, antiradical and antifungal activities in orange and apple juices. Food Chemistry 2011;126 1749–1758.

[65] Vulic J, Canadanović-Brunet J, Cetković G, Tumbas V, Djilas S, Cetojević-Simin D, Canadanović V. Antioxidant and cell growth activities of beet root pomace extracts. Journal of Functional Foods 2012;4 670–678.

[66] Kallel F, Driss D, Chaari F, Belghith L, Bouaziz F, Ghorbel R, Chaabouni SE. Garlic (*Allium sativum* L.) husk waste as a potential source of phenolic compounds: Influence of extracting solvents on its antimicrobial andantioxidant properties. Industrial Crops and Products 2014;62 34–41.

[67] Tutin TG, Heywood HV, Burges NA, Valentine DH, Walters SM, Webb DA. Diapensiaceae to Myoporaceae. In Flora Euroapea, vol. 3. Cambridge, United Kingdom: Cambridge University Press; 2001.

[68] European Medicines Agency. *Community Herbal Monograph on Thymus vulgaris L. and Thymus zygis L., herba.* http://www.ema.europa.eu/ema/index.jsp?curl=pages/medicines/herbal/medicines/herbal_med_000029.jsp&mid=WC0b01ac058001fa1d (Accessed 15 December 2014).

[69] *European Pharmacopeia.* 2002. 4th edition. Strasbourg Cedex: Council of Europe, Vol. 2.8.12: 183–184.

[70] Lakic N, Mimica-Dukic N, Isak J, Bozin B. Antioxidant properties of *Galium verum* L. (Rubiaceae) extracts. Central European Journal of Biology 2010;5(3) 331–337.

[71] Jia Z, Tang M, Wu J. The determination of flavonoids content in mulbery and scavenging effect on superoxide radicals. Food Chemistry 1999;64 555–599.

[72] Božin B, Kladar N, Grujić N, Anačkov G, Samojlik I, Gavarić N, Srđenović Čonić B. Impact of origin and biological source on chemical composition, anticholinesterase and antioxidant properties of some St. John' Wort species (*Hypericum spp.*, Hypericaceae) from Central Balkans. Molecules 2013;18 11733–11750.

[73] Misan A, Mimica-Dukic N, Mandic A, Sakac M, Milovanovic I, Sedej I. Development of a rapid resolution HPLC method for the separation and determination of 17 phenolic compounds in crude plant extracts. Central European Journal of Chemistry 2011;9(1) 133–142.

[74] Klančnik A, Piskernik S, Jeršek B, SmoleMožina S. Evaluation of diffusion and dilution methods to determine the antibacterial activity of plant extracts. Journal of Microbiological Methods 2010;81 121–126.

[75] Valgas C, de Souza SM, Smânia EFA, Smânia JA. Screening methods to determine antibacterial activity of natural products. Brazilian Journal of Microbiology 2007;38 369–380.

[76] Das K, Tiwari RKS, Shrivastava DK. Techniques for evaluation of medicinal plant products as antimicrobial agent: Current methods and future trends. Journal of Medicinal Plants Research 2010; 4(2) 104–111.

[77] CLSI (NCCLS) Methods for Dilution Antimicrobial Susceptibility Tests for Bacteria that Grow Aerobically: Approved Standard 23. National Committee for Clinical Laboratory Standards, Wayne, PA, USA; 2003.

[78] Grare M, Fontanay S, Cornil C, Finance C, Duval ER. Tetrazolium salts for MIC determination in microplates: Why? Which salt to select? How? Journal of Microbiological Methods 2008;75 156–159.

[79] Ellof JN. A sensitive and quick microplate method to determine the minimal inhibitory concentration of plant extracts for bacteria. Planta Medica 1998;64 711–713.

[80] Klančnik A, Guzej B, HadolinKolnar M, Abramovič H, SmoleMožina S. *In vitro* antimicrobial and antioxidant activity of commercial rosemary extract formulations. Journal of Food Protection 2009;72 1744–1752.

[81] Scudiero DA, Shoemaker RH, Paull KD, Monks A, Tierney S, Nofziger TH, Currens MJ, Seniff D, Boyd MR. Evaluation of a soluble tetrazolium/formazan assay for cell growth and drug sensitivity using human and other tumor cell lines. Cancer Research 1988;48 4827–4833.

[82] Rinner B, Kretschmer N, Knausz H, Mayer A, Boechzelt H, Hao XJ, Heubl G, Efferth T, Schaider H, Bauer R. A petrol ether extract of the roots of *Onosmapaniculatum* induces cell death in a caspase dependent manner. Journal of Ethnopharmacology 2010;129 182–188.

[83] Herodež SS, Hadolin M, Škerget M, Knez Ž. Solvent extraction study of antioxidants from balm (*Melissa officinalis* L.) leaves. Food Chemistry 2003;80(2) 275–282.

[84] Negi PS. Plant extracts for the control of bacterial growth: Efficacy, stability, and safety for food application. International Journal of Food Microbiology 2012;156 7–17.

[85] Mimica-Dukic N, Bozin B. *Mentha* L. Species (Lamiaceae) as promising sources of bioactive secondary metabolites. Current Pharmaceutical Design 2008;14(29) 3141–3150.

[86] Sohn HY, Son KH, Kwon GS, Kang SS. Antimicrobial and cytotoxic activity of 18 prenylated flavonoids isolated from medicinal plants: *Morus alba* L., *Morus mongolica* Schneider, *Broussnetia papyrifera* (L.) Vent., *Sophora flavescens* Ait and *Echinosophora koreensis* Nakai. Phytomedicine 2004;11 666–672.

[87] Moure A, Cruz JM, Franco D, Domínguez JM, Sinieiro J, Domínguez H, Núñez MJ, Parajó JC. Natural antioxidants from residual sources. Food Chemistry 2001;72 145–171.

[88] Lakic N. Postdistillation waste of aromatic plants as a potential source for pharmaceutical industry. PhD thesis. University of Novi Sad; 2013.

[89] EFSA, The European Union report on trends and sources of zoonoses, zoonotic agents and food-borne outbreaks in 2011, EFSA J. 11 (2013) 3129.

[90] Kaur K, Kumar V, Sharma AK, Gupta GK. Isoxazoline containing natural products as anticancer agents: A review. European Journal of Medicinal Chemistry 2014;77 121–133.

[91] Garamukulya Y, Abou-Elella F, Wamunyokoli F, Aei-Shemy H. Phytochemical screening, anti-oxidant activity and in vitro anticancer potential of ethanolic and water leaves extracts of Annona muricata (Graviola) Asian Pacific Journal of Tropical Medicine 2014;7(suppl 1) S355–S363.

[92] Smole Možina S, Kurinčič M, Klančnik A, Mavri A. *Campylobacter* and its multi-resistance in the food chain. Trends in Food Science & Technology 2011;22 91–98.

[93] Voljč M, Levart A., Žgur S, Salobir J. The effect of α-tocopherol, sweet chestnut wood extract and their combination on oxidative stress in vivo and the oxidative stability of meat in broilers. British Poultry Science 2013;54(1) 144–156.

[94] Dalle Zotte A, Cullere M, Sartori A, Szendrő Z, Kovàcs M, Giaccone V, Dal Bosco A. Dietary Spirulina (*Arthrospira platensis*) and Thyme (*Thymus vulgaris*) supplementation to growing rabbits: Effects on raw and cooked meat quality, nutrient true retention and oxidative stability. Meat Science 2014;98(2) 94–103.

[95] Dal Bosco A, Gerencsér Zs, Szendrő Zs, Mugnai C, Cullere M, Kovàcs M, Ruggeri S, Mattioli S, Castellini C, Dalle Zotte A. Effect of dietary supplementation of Spirulina (*Arthrospira platensis*) and Thyme (*Thymus vulgaris*) on rabbit meat appearance, oxidative stability and fatty acid profile during retail display. Meat Science 2014;96(1) 114–119.

Chapter 7

Phytopharmaceutical Studies of Selected Medicinal Plants Subjected to Abiotic Elicitation (Stress) in Industrial Area

Sr. Prema Kumari Jonnada, Louis Jesudas and Varaprasad Bobbarala

Additional information is available at the end of the chapter

http://dx.doi.org/10.5772/61891

Abstract

Plants are a source of large amount of drugs comprising antispasmodics, emetic, Anti-cancer, anti microbial and anticancer activities etc. A large number of the plants are claimed to possess the antibiotic properties in the traditional system and today they are extensively used by the people and the metal Components in the plants grown in polluted area seemingly increase the concentration of phytochemicals. Recent times the flora and fauna of any region is directly or indirectly exposed to the all types pollutants which may result into adverse effects rarely the metal pollutants may trigger the production of phytochemicals. The present study deals with Industrial pollution of the area selected for study, metal up take, and their effect on phytochemical, anti-microbial and anticancer activities that explore the research on five medicinal plants namely *Adhatoda vasica, Eucalyptus globulus, Hyptis suaveolens, Ricinus communis* and *Tinospora cordifolia* that thrive well and grow luxuriantly in industrial polluted area and the same five plants from natural area of Visakhapatnam District. The aim of this study is to analyze the effect of Metal elements on phytochemical productivity and antimicrobial and anticancer activity of these medicinal plants. Metal analysis is done ICP-MS (PerkinElmer Sciex Instrument, model ELAN DRC II, USA). Alkaloids, flavanoids, terpenoids and phenols screening is done in solvents Hexane, Chloroform and methanol and checked for antimicrobial activity and anti-cancer activity of *Eucalyptus globulus* and *Tinospora cordifolia* were determined by XTT assay on MCF-7 cell lines. The results are discussed in comparison of Natural with pollutant grown plants. The plants that showed better production of phytochemicals due to the presence of metal elements could be recommended to phytopharmaceutical industries as they comparatively showed better production of phytochemicals further proposing a definite way to eliminate toxic metals from them.

Keywords: Abiotic Elicitation, Industrial Area, Medicinal Plants

1. Introduction

The stupendous glory of India is unparalleled and unmatched. No other country, worldwide, can compare itself to this glory of India. Whether it is the magnificent waterfalls and sacred rivers, lush canopies and verdant valleys, or the varied and rich flora and fauna, India has it all including ecological islands, such as Visakhapatnam in Andhra Pradesh, which harbours endemic plants [1]. There are more than two thousand plant species acknowledged to have medicinal value in the traditional Asian system of medicine. This health-giving store, India is blessed to have experienced every creation of "Mother Nature."

The Eastern Ghats properties of medicinal plants are due to the presence of various complex chemical substances of different composition which occur as secondary metabolites [2]. They are grouped as alkaloids, glycosides, corticosteroids, coumarin, flavonoids, and essential oils. Flavonoids are chemical compounds that are active against microorganisms. They have been found in vitro to be effective antimicrobial substances against a wide array of microorganisms [3].

Phytochemicals are naturally occurring, biologically active chemical compounds that protect plants against bacteria, fungi, and viruses and have potential benefits for health. The presence of certain types of phytochemicals in some plants can act as a natural defense system providing protection against such things as attacks from insects and grazing animals. In contrast, other plants produce phytochemicals that provide colour, aroma, and flavor and improve immune function. They stop toxic substances from becoming carcinogens in your body, protect and repair your DNA, reduce inflammation, normalize hormone levels, and slow the growth of cancer cells. Phytochemicals have recently become of great interest owing to their versatile applications.

Medicinal plants are the richest bioresource of drugs for traditional systems of medicine, modern medicines, nutraceuticals, food supplements, folk medicines, pharmaceutical intermediates, and chemical entities for synthetic drugs [4]. Presently, herbal remedies are preferred due to less or no side effects for many diseases, and due to financial constraints [5]. Despite enormous developments in synthetic medicines, several other diseases have grown due to their harmful side effects after prolonged use [6, 7]. Since the dawn of history, plants have played an important role in the treatment of human ailments. Over 50% of all modern clinical drugs are of natural origin and natural products play an important role in drug development programs in the pharmaceutical industry. Herbal drugs have gained importance in recent years because of their efficacy and cost-effectiveness [8]. The plants which have been selected for medicinal use over thousands of years constitute the most obvious choice of examining the current search for therapeutically effective new drugs such as anticancer drugs [9], antimicrobial drugs [10], and antihepatotoxic compounds [11, 12]. According to the World Health Organization (WHO), medicinal plants are the best source to obtain a variety of drugs. About 80% of individuals from developed countries use traditional medicines, which have compounds derived from medicinal plants.

However, such plants should be investigated to better understand their properties, safety, and efficiency. Knowledge of the chemical constituents of plants is desirable because such information will be of value for synthesis of complex chemical substances [13, 14, 16].

http://dx.doi.org/10.5772/61891

These medicinal plants that are rich biosources of several drugs in the treatment and prevention of many diseases are constantly exposed to pollutants directly or indirectly. Especially plants growing in industrial area (surrounded by oil refinery) are subjected to a range of pollutants (external factors) that may adversely affect the growth and development of cultivated plants and crops. These factors may impose an abiotic stress on medicinal plants too, which may alter metabolic profiles and developmental trajectories and thereby induce the production of various secondary metabolites. This in turn assists the plant to adapt varied environmental changes.

In the area selected for my study, the sources of pollutants are mainly industries. Taking into consideration the above mentioned three factors:

1. The promising effects of phytochemicals and antimicrobial activity

2. The negative effect of pollutants on medicinal plants and, in turn, on human health,

3. The interesting and contrasting positive role of metal elements in increasing and eliciting the secondary metabolites and their antimicrobial and therapeutic activity; we have selected two areas of research interest in the Eastern Ghats.

Visakhapatnam in Andhra Pradesh, the area of my study, popularly known as Vizag, is a booming industrial city on the east coast of India. It is located on the eastern shore of India nestled among the Eastern Ghats' Hill Ranges and facing the Bay of Bengal on the East. It is a port city with the biggest ship-building yard in India and is also the headquarters of the Eastern Naval Command. The district presents two distinct geographic divisions. A strip of land along the coast called the plain division, having an altitude not more than 75 m and a hilly area of Eastern Ghats flanking it on the North West called agency division having an altitude of 900 m. Vizag supports a rich diversity of plant wealth due to its annual rainfall.

The first area of my study is a large residential area at the lower altitude of Eastern Ghats Malkapuram in Visakhapatnam, where there are more than fourteen major hazardous industries, among which seven are present in the Malkapuram cluster, namely, HPCL (R), HPCL (T), IOCL (T), LPG bolting plant, CFL, APCL, and BPCL. The soil and medicinal plants that are thriving well and have luxuriant growth in the Malkapuram cluster were chosen as the source in the industrially polluted zone. The area may be polluted with various heavy metals such as cadmium, lead, copper, manganese, cobalt, nickel, aluminum, zinc, iron, chromium, etc. Owing to the low-quality fuel that is processed in refineries, these substances exert abiotic stress on the plant species that inhabits those areas. The plants grown in natural conditions may have less or no abiotic stress [16] (Plate 1).

The second area of my study is the Paderu division of Visakhapatnam district, the higher altitude zone in the hilly tracts of Eastern Ghats of Andhra Pradesh. It has the second highest tribal population in Andhra Pradesh. The tribal people of this division largely depend on herbal medicines, plant products for primary health care, and their daily life [17]. This area is considered to be free from industries and therefore the biosphere in this zone is less polluted.

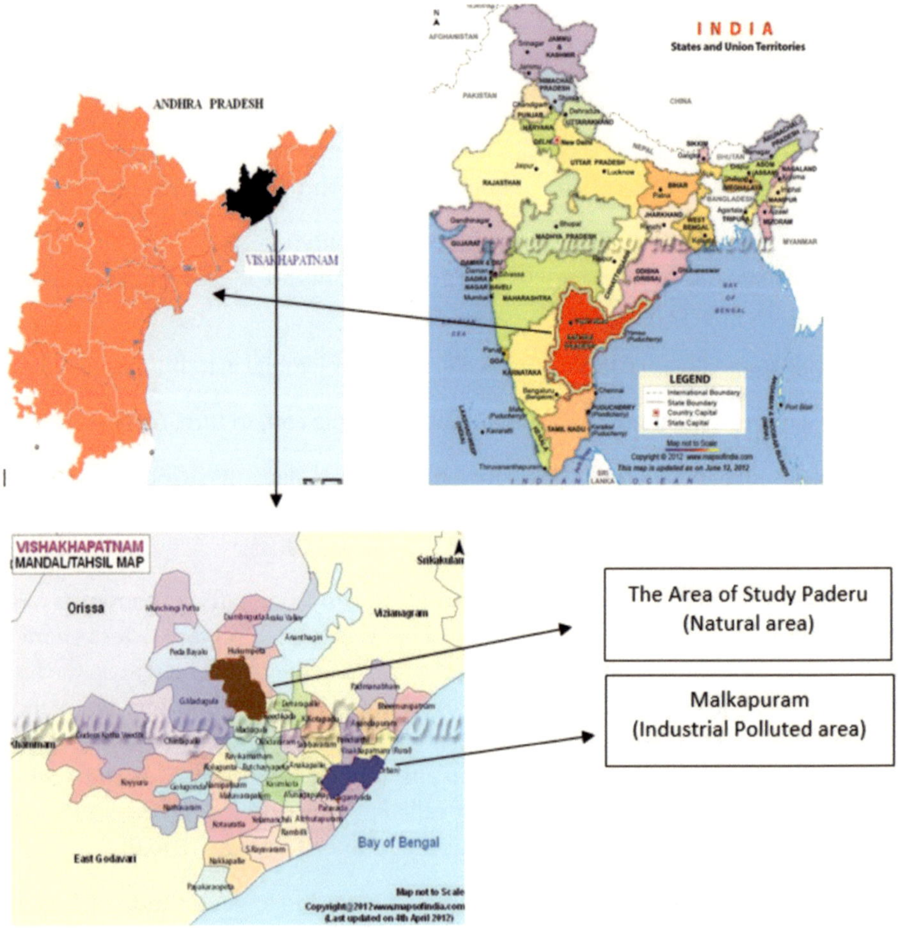

Plate 1. The map of Visakhapatnam in Andhra Pradesh and the areas selected for study.

1.1. Justification

Plants, when exposed to unfavorable environments, such as water deficit, chilling, heat stress, oxygen deficiency, and air pollution, result in some degree of stress and express only a fraction of the plants' genetic potential. Plants adapt to unfavorable conditions through genetically determined stress resistance [18]. Plants grown in a given habitat are exposed to various abiotic stresses that may have significant effects on their growth and productivity. Environmental factors such as light, water, as well as salinity are important variables affecting phytochemical production in plants [19]. Abiotic stresses will affect the pathways involved in the biosynthesis of the 3 principal groups of secondary metabolites: terpenes, phenolics, and nitrogen-containing compounds. These compounds serve as the plants' defenses against herbivores and pathogens, as attractants for pollinators and seed-dispersing animals, and assist with absorbing harmful ultraviolet radiation or reducing the growth of competing plants among others [20]. Owing to their biological activity, secondary metabolites are used commercially as insecticides, fungicides, pharmaceuticals, fragrances, flavorings, medicinal drugs, and industrial materials.

Oxidative stress induced by heavy metals triggers signaling pathways that affect the production of specific plant metabolites [21]. Similar observations have been noted by several research groups [22]. However, high levels of heavy metal contamination in medicinal or other plants may suppress secondary metabolite production. Alternatively, the presence of heavy metals in medicinal plants may stimulate the production of bioactive compounds in many plant species. In addition, trace element levels have become of prime importance for both the clinical diagnosis and curing of different diseases [23]. Trace elements play a vital role in medicinal plants and are therefore responsible for their medicinal properties [24].

A large number of the plants that reportedly possess antibiotic and antioxidant properties in the traditional system are today extensively used by the people, and the metal components in plants grown in polluted areas seemingly increase the concentration of phytochemicals. In recent times, the flora and fauna of any region have been directly or indirectly exposed to all types of pollutants, which may result in adverse effects where rarely the metal pollutants may trigger the production of phytochemicals. Industrial activities have become a threat to medicinal plants as they release metallic compounds to the atmosphere, leading to heavy metal accumulation in crops and medicinal plants. Large residential areas, especially near the industrial belt, are contaminated by heavy metals that mainly originate from industrial activity in the Malkapuram cluster—the area of our study. However, elevated levels of both essential and nonessential heavy metals pose a serious threat for human health and agriculture.

Contrary to many views, the metal components in the medicinal plants grown in polluted areas seemingly increase the concentration of phytochemicals.

Around the world, it is estimated that 9 million new cases of cancer are diagnosed every year and over 4.5 million people die of disease. In India, 7 lakh cases and over 3.5 lakhs of people die of cancer every year, and 2.3 lakhs of new cases are tobacco related. The leading cancer among males is pharyngeal cancer, which accounts for 14.1% of total cancers, whereas the leading cancer among females is cervical cancer, which accounts for 26.7% of cancers, this is followed by breast cancer, which accounts for 16.6% [25, 26]. As per the statistics news of the WHO, the number of people being diagnosed with cancer in the world has leaped to more than 14 million each year.

India is the first of the emerging economics to join the IARC in 2006, and is an active participating state of the global cancer research agency. In India, around 5, 55, 000 people died of cancer in 2010. According to estimates published in *Lancet*, of which 45% were deaths from breast cancer [27]. Breast cancer in urban Indian women is 25–30 and the age is adjusted to 30–35 and the new cases 100, 000–125, 000 breast cancer cases every year in India [28].

A number of undecided side effects that occur during chemotherapy can be reduced by using plant-derived products in cancer treatments. Various active compounds derived from medicinal plants have been assisting for their efficacy and tolerability and treatment of breast cancer. The present work is an attempt to find out metal analysis, phytochemical, antimicrobial activity, and cytotoxicity of crude extracts of selected medicinal plants particularly *Eucalyptus globulus* and *Tinospora cordifolia* on MCF-7 breast cancer cell lines.

2. Aims and objectives

The present study was aimed to identify and collect the plants that are thriving well in both industrial and natural areas and their comparative analysis of metal, phytochemical, antimicrobial, and anticancer activities.

This research details the uptake of metals by various medicinal plants grown in polluted and natural sources and their effect on phytochemical, antimicrobial, and anticancer activities. The study includes 5 pairs of plants (for a total of 10 samples). *Adhatoda vasica*, Nees, *Hyptis suaveolens*, (L.)Poit, *E. globulus*, Labill., *Ricinus communis* Linn., and *T. cordifolia*, Meirs. These plants that are under metal stress may trigger secondary metabolites of pharmacological importance, which may be a boon to the pharmacological industries to exploit their phytochemical nature and in turn become beneficial to mankind.

Therefore, the present study was undertaken with the following objectives:

- Identification, selection and collection of some medicinal plants that are grown abundantly and luxuriantly in both natural and industrial areas
- Metal analysis of selected medicinal plants and soils from both areas and their comparative study
- Qualitative phytochemical analysis, and estimation of total phenols and antibacterial activity of the medicinal plants that are grown in natural and industrial areas
- The comparative study on the effect of metals on phytochemicals and their antibacterial activity
- Role of phytochemicals on MCF-7 breast cancer cell lines
- Finally, to recommend those plants which elicit phytochemical, antimicrobial, and anticancer activities to the pharmaceuticals for further detailed study and for the usage conformity by the experts.

3. Collection of plant material

In the present study, an initial survey was done in polluted areas that were previously mentioned and found to be dominated by about 20 plant species. Out of these 20 plant species, 10 were screened and selected based on their luxuriant growth and medicinal properties. Furthermore, we restricted our study to 5 plants (Table 1) to make our analysis more concrete. The same species of plant materials were collected from polluted areas and from natural areas

http://dx.doi.org/10.5772/61891

of Visakhapatnam district, Andhra Pradesh, India. All plants were screened for their metal elements and, among them, five plants from each area were selected for qualitative and quantitative phytochemical analysis and antimicrobial and anticancer studies. The collected materials were washed thoroughly under running tap water and finally with sterile distilled water, then the materials were air-dried on a sterile blotter under shade to constant weight for a period of 45 days.

S No.	Plant name	Family
1	*A. vasica,* Nees	Acanthaceae
2	*E. globulus,* Labill	Myrtaceae
3	*H. suaveolens,* (L.) Poit.	Labiatae
4	*R. communis,* Linn.	Euphorbiaceae
5	*T. cordifolia,* Miers	Menispermaceae

Table 1. List of medicinal plants selected from industrially polluted and natural areas of Visakhapatnam district

The collected plant specimens were identified with the help of *Flora of the Presidency of Madras* [29] and *Flora of Visakhapatnam* by Subba Rao [30] and *Flora of Srikakulam* by Sheshagiri and Sreeramulu [31], and they were confirmed by the taxonamist Mr. Ramesh of Andhra University, Visakhapatnam. The selected plant materials (Plates 2 and 3) are given with short descriptions.

3.1. *A. vasica,* Nees

A. vasica, Nees belongs to the family called Acanthaceae. All plains Districts, perhaps wild in the *N. Circars,* elsewhere cultivated as a hedge plant and runs wild near villages. A dense shrub with a foetid scent, the flowers are white with the throat barred with red or yellow. The leaves are used in native medicine, and an infusion can be used as an insecticide. Vern. Hind. Arusha; Ur. Basung; Tel. Addasaram; Tam. Adatodai [32] (Plate 2a).

3.2. *E. globulus,* Labill.

E. globulus, Labill. belongs to the family called Myrtaceae, largely grown in forests on the Nilgiris and other hills of the W. Ghats and frequently found self-sown. The Blue Gum is a lofty tree with very grey young leaves and narrow, green, linear-lanceolate, curved, vertically hanging old leaves; white, rather large flowers, and ribose capsule, all parts very aromatic with a valuable essential oil which is largely extracted. The bark is grey, with deciduous the outer layers; wood grey with darker streak, moderately hard, used in building but most especially for fuel [33] (Plate 2b).

3.3. *H. suaveolens,* (L.) Poit.

H. suaveolens Poit. belongs to the family of Labiatae. Most plains Districts, on roadsides and waste ground, introduced from Tropical America and runs wild. A tall, sweet-smelling herb with tetragonal hispid stems, ovate, cordate, denticulate leaves reaching 4.5 in. long and small blue flowers, the fruiting calyx campanulate and ribbed with 5 arista teeth. Vern. Hind. Wilayati tulasi [32] (Plate 2c).

3.4. *R. communis*, Linn.

R. communis, Linn. belongs to the family called Euphorbiaceae. Cultivated and found running wild in the fields and gardens, by roadsides, and on wastelands. The castor-oil plant is often almost a small tree with a thin greyish-brown bark and soft white wood. It is cultivated for the oil which is extracted from the seeds and used for burning, as a lubricant and in medicine. Vern. Hind, Arend; Tam, Sitta-munuk; Tel. Amadam; Kan. Haralu [33] (Plate 3a).

3.5. *T. cordifolia*, Miers

T. cordifolia, Miers belongs to the family called Menispermaceae. A climbing shrub with succulent stems, the bark is papery at first then corky, leaves glabrous, flowers yellow, on nodes on the old wood; drupes red and sessile; endocarp with a few isolated tubercles or smooth. It is grown in forests and among trees in almost all districts. Vern. Hind. Goluncha; Tel. Tippa tiga; Tam. Chintil [32] (Plate 3b).

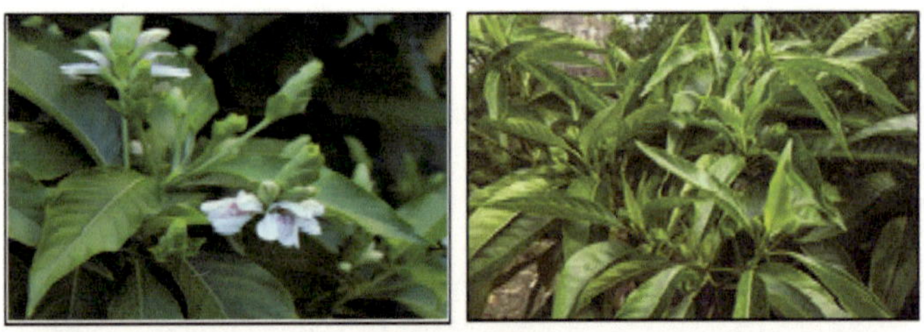

(a) *Adhatoda vasica, Nees*

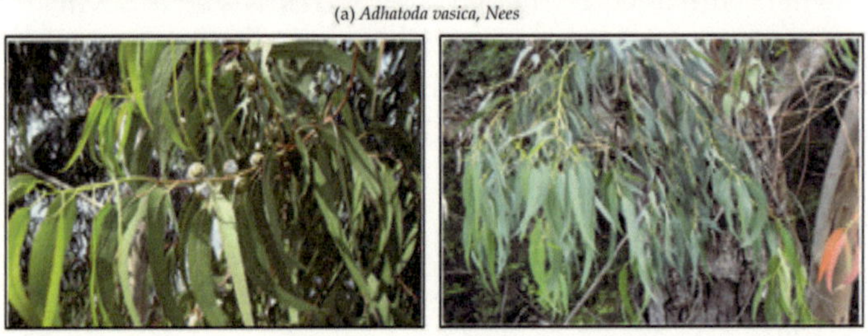

(b) *Eucalyptus globulus, Labill*

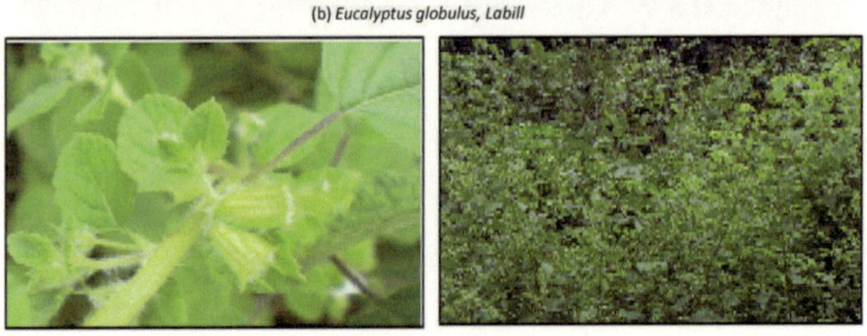

(c) *Hyptis sua veolens, Poit*

Plate 2. Medicinal plants selected for the present study.

http://dx.doi.org/10.5772/61891

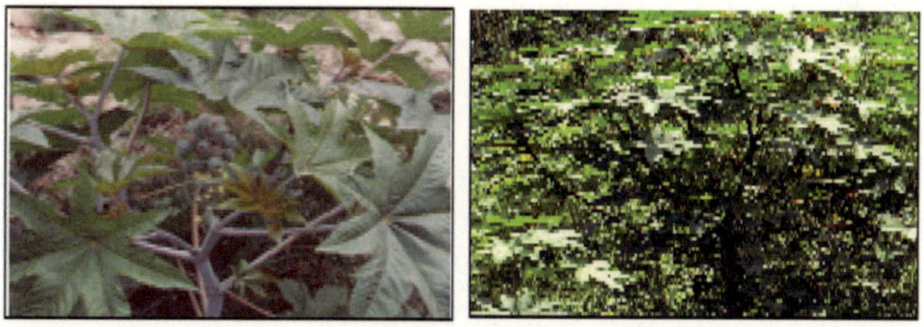

(a) *Ricinus communis*, Linn

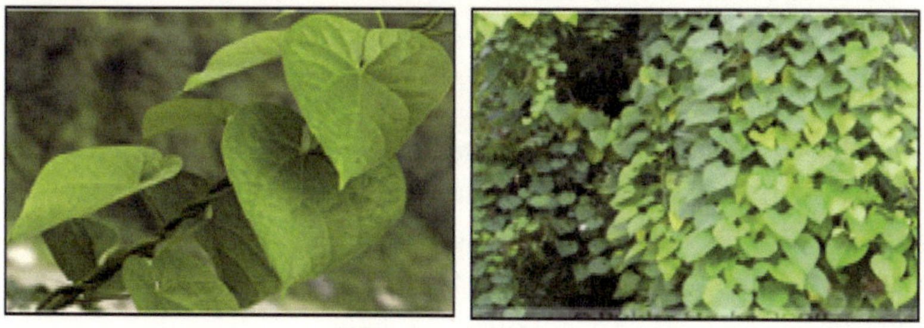

(b) *Tinospora cordifolia*, Miers

Plate 3. Medicinal Plants Selected for the Present Study

3.6. Experimental: Metal analysis

3.6.1. Instrumentation

A Perkin Elmer SCIEX model Elan® DRC II ICP-MS (Ontario, Canada) at CSIR-National Geophysical Research Institute, Hyderabad, was used throughout for trace elemental analysis of plant and soil samples. The sample introduction system consisted of a standard Meinhard® nebulizer with a cyclonic spray chamber.

3.6.2. Materials

A hot plate with digital temperature controller with a maximum temperature of 250°C was used for digestion. Teflon® beakers were thoroughly cleaned, soaked in 1:1 HNO_3 for 6 h, and thoroughly rinsed with Milli-Q water were used for digestion. Thoroughly acid-cleaned 100 and 250 ml standard flasks were used for volume make up. Whattman filter paper no. 42 was used for filtration purposes.

3.6.3. Determination of trace metals in soil

About 0.05 g soil samples were weighed and taken in a clean PTFE Teflon® beaker. Each sample was moistened with a few drops of water. Then, 10 ml of the acid mixture containing a 7:3:1 ratio of HF, HNO_3, and $HClO_4$ was added to each beaker and the sample swirled until completely moistened. The beakers were covered with lids and the samples were left standing overnight after adding 5 ml of ^{103}Rh (1 µg/ml) as an internal standard. The next day, the beakers were heated on a hot plate at 220°C for about 1 h, after which the lids were removed, and the contents evaporated to near-dryness. The evaporation process was repeated after adding 5 ml of the above acid mixture in each case. Finally, the residue was dissolved by gently heating in 20 ml of 1:1 HNO_3. Clear solutions were obtained for all samples. After cooling to room temperature, the volume was made up to 250 ml, and these final solutions were stored in polyethylene bottles. The concentrations of different metals in these solutions were analyzed by ICP-MS. International geochemical standards SO-1 and SO-2 were used for calibration as well as to check the accuracy and precision.

3.6.4. Determination of trace metals in plants

Open acid digestion method was followed for the determination of metal concentration, wherein representative samples of dried plant tissues (approximately ~0.5 g) were taken in Teflon® beakers and 30 ml conc. HNO_3 were added in each. They were heated on a hot plate (~100°C) for 2 h keeping the lids. At the boiling stage, about 4–5 ml of H_2O_2 was added dropwise and heated further and the volume was reduced to about 10 ml. During this entire process, all organic material gets oxidized and the inorganic contents are extracted into the solution. To this, 5 ml of 1 µg/g Rh solution was added to act as an internal standard and the solution was transferred to a 250 ml volumetric flask and diluted to 250 ml with Milli-Q® water. The solution was analyzed by ICP-MS for trace elements.

3.7. Phytochemical screening

3.7.1. Solvent extraction of plant material

The completely shade-dried plant materials were ground into fine powder using an electric blender. The powdered plant material was subjected to successive solvent extraction taking from nonpolar to polar solvents like hexane, chloroform, and methanol, 70 g of powdered plant material was subjected to soxhlet extraction for 8 h with 300 ml of the various solvents. Each time before employing the solvent of higher polarity marc was dried. The extracts obtained were later kept for evaporation to remove the excessive solvents and brought to complete dryness over a water bath to yield the crude extracts. These extracts were collected, labeled, and stored at 4°C for further study.

3.7.2. Qualitative analysis of phytochemicals (Brindha et al. 1981)

The extract was tested for the presence of bioactive compounds by using the following standard methods given by Brindha et al. [34].

a. **Detection of alkaloids:** Extract (0.5 g) was dissolved in 10 ml of dilute HCl (0.1 N) and filtered. The filtrate was used to test for the presence of alkaloids. Mayer's test/Mayer's reagent: 1.358 g of mercuric chloride in 60 ml of water and 5 g of KI in 10 ml water. Mix the 2 solutions and dilute to 100 ml water. Filtrate was treated with Mayer's reagent. The formation of yellow cream precipitate indicates the presence of alkaloids.

b. **Detection of terpenoids**: Five milliliters of each extract was mixed in 2 ml of chloroform, and concentrated H_2SO_4 (3 ml) was carefully added to form a layer. A reddish brown colouration of the interface was formed to show positive results for the presence of terpenoids.

c. **Detection of saponins**: The ability of saponins to produce frothing in aqueous solutions was used as a screening test for the sample. Dried extract (0.5 g) was shaken with water in a test tube; froth which persist upon warming was taken as evidence for the presence of saponins. Honeycomb froth indicated the presence of saponins.

d. **Detection of tannins**: To the extract, 1% of gelatin solution containing sodium chloride was added. Formation of white precipitate indicates the presence of tannins.

e. **Detection of phenols:** The extract was treated with 3 to 4 drops of 1% $FeCl_3$ solution. Formation of bluish black colour indicates phenols.

f. **Detection of flavonoids:** Extracts were treated with a few drops of sodium hydroxide solution. Formation of intense yellow colour, which becomes colourless upon the addition of dilute acid, indicates the presence of flavonoids.

3.7.3. Quantitative analysis of phytochemicals

a. **Determination of total flavonoid content using Swain and Hills method [35].** Preparation of standard and test solutions: The plant extract (50 mg) was dissolved separately in 50 ml of methanol. These solutions were serially diluted with methanol to get lower dilutions. Phloroglucinol (50 mg) was dissolved in 50 ml of distilled water. It was serially diluted with water to get lower dilutions.

Protocol for flavonoid content estimation: 0.2 ml of extract was taken in a test tube and the final volume was adjusted to 2.0 ml with distilled water. To this, 4.0 ml of vanillin reagent was added rapidly. Exactly after 15 min, absorbance was recorded at 500 nm against a blank. The unknown was read from the standard curves using different concentrations of phloroglucinol.

b. **Protocol for total phenol content estimation.** Total natural phenols of plant extracts were determined using a Folin–Ciocalteu assay with minor modifications [36]. A test tube containing either 500 µl of standard solutions of gallic acid (50, 25, 12.5, 6.25, 3.125, 1.5625, and 0.78125 µg/ml) or crude extracts (diluted 400-fold with distilled deionized water) was prepared, 500 µl of 10% Folin–Ciocalteu's phenol reagent (in DDW) was added into each test tube and mixed. After 20 min, 350 µl of 1 M Na_2CO_3 solution was added into the mixture. After incubation for 20 min at room temperature, the absorbance was determined at 750 nm against the blank prepared in parallel (500 µl of DDW + 500 µl of 10% FC reagent + 350 µl of 1 M Na_2CO_3 solution). The results expressed as gallic acid equivalents from the standard curve.

3.8. Antimicrobial activity

3.8.1. *In vitro antimicrobial assay*

The antimicrobial activity of the hexane, chloroform and methanol extracts of each sample was evaluated by using well diffusion method or cup plate method modified by Olurinola, which is the most widely used type for identifying antimicrobial activity, and exploited the diffusion of antimicrobial compounds through agar media to demonstrate the inhibition of bacteria and fungi [37, 38].

3.8.2. *Collection of microbial cultures*

Based on common diseases in human beings, 8 pathogenic species were selected to perform the antimicrobial action of test samples. The names of the cultures are listed in Table 2. All the cultures were collected from TRIMS, Visakhapatnam in Andhra Pradesh.

ID No.	ID Name	Morphology
MTCC 96	*Staphylococcus aureus*	Gram-positive facultative anaerobic, grape-like clusters
MTCC 430	*Bacillus cereus*	Gram-positive large endospore former
MTCC 2274	*Bacillus subtilis*	Gram-positive rod-shaped, motile, peritrichous flagella, aerobic
MTCC 439	*Enterococcus faecalis*	Gram-positive lactic acid bacteria of the phylum Firmicutes
MTCC 7162	*Klebsiella pneumonia*	Gram-negative bacilli, shorter and thicker rods about 1–2 mm encapsulated (thick caps)
MTCC 1457	*Shigella boydii* (serogroup C)	Gram-negative bacilli, short rods measuring from 0.5 to 1.3 m, nonvolatile, non–spore-forming, and noncapsulated
MTCC 443	*Escherichia coli*	Gram-negative, straight rod measuring 1.3 × 0.4 to 0.7 mm, motile capsulated
MTCC 3072	*Candida albicans*	Diploid fungus that grows both as yeast and filamentous cell, Chlamydosporous

Table 2. List of microorganisms used for antimicrobial activity with the diseases they cause

3.8.3. *Media used for antimicrobial assay*

For bioassay studies, the media used was Mueller–Hinton agar. The addition of the agar to the medium creates a solid matrix and by avoiding any significant mixing, the culture is good for inoculating microbes on the surface of the medium as required for isolation of pure cultures.

Composition of Mueller–Hinton agar medium

Beef infusion; 300.0 g/l, Casein, 17.5 gm/l

Agar; 17.0 g/l, Starch, 1.5 g/l

3.8.4. Preparation of culture

A loop-full of clinically tested precultures was reconstituted in sterile peptone water to produce a suspension of microbial cells.

3.8.5. Preparation of media and plates for agar diffusion method

This assay was performed using two methods: agar disc diffusion and agar well diffusion. In these two methods, the agar well diffusion assay was used to screen for antimicrobial activity of the hexane chloroform and the methanolic extracts of different plant species. To prepare the media, for each organism, it requires 20 plates of MTT agar for 500 ml of distilled water; 19.5 g of MH agar was weighed and dissolved in a conical flask. Then, it was autoclaved at 15 lbs. pressure at 121°C for 20 min. After sterilization, media was aseptically distributed into sterile 6-in. diameter petri plates and allowed to solidify at room temperature for about 10 min and then kept in a refrigerator for 30 min. After solidification, using a sterile cotton swab, each microbial culture was spread uniformly onto the surface of the agar plates from culture containing approximately 105 CFU/ml of each organism for 24 h slant culture in aseptic conditions. The most widely used type of identifying antimicrobial activity is the diffusion method, which exploits the diffusion of antimicrobial compounds through the agar media to demonstrate inhibition of bacteria. The assay was performed by using a well-plate method. After inoculation of culture into each petri plate, a well borer of 5 mm diameter was properly sterilized by flame and used to make 6 uniform wells in each petri plate. These wells were labeled based on the microbes and plant extract used. To determine the potential of plant extracts, they were diluted up to 100 mg/ml of DMSO solution. And from three solvent extract dilutions, 40 μl was introduced into wells, respectively, and allowed to diffuse for 45 min. The plates were incubated at 37°C for 24 h. After proper incubation, the zones of inhibition were measured with a ruler. Results were noted and presented.

3.9. Anticancer activity

3.9.1. Cell culture

Human cancer cell lines used in this study were procured from the National Centre for Cell Science, Pune. All cells were grown in minimal essential medium (MEM, GIBCO) supplemented with 4.5 g/L glucose, antibiotics (benzyl penicillin, 50 units/m; streptomycin, 50 μg/ml, and amphotericin-B, 50 μg/ml), 2 mM L-glutamine and 5% fetal bovine serum (FBS) (growth medium) at 37°C in 5% CO_2 incubator.

3.9.2. XTT assay

The biochemical procedure is based on the activity of mitochondrial enzymes, which are inactivated shortly after cell death. This method was found to be very efficient in assessing the viability of cells. A colorimetric method based on the tetrazolium salt, XTT, was first described [39]. In brief, the trypsinized cells from T-25 flask were seeded in each well of 96-well flat-bottomed tissue culture plate at a density of 5×10^3 cells/well in growth medium and cultured at 37°C in 5% CO_2 to adhere. After 24 h of incubation, the supernatant was discarded and the cells were pretreated with growth medium and subsequently mixed with different concentrations of test compounds (12.5, 25, 50, 100, and 200 μg/ml) in triplicate to achieve a final volume of 100 μl and then cultured for 48 h. The compound was prepared as 1.0 mg/ml concentration stock solutions in DMSO. Culture medium and solvent were used as controls. Each well then received 50 μl of fresh XTT (0.9 mg/ml in RPMI along with XTT activator reagent) followed by incubation for 2 h at 37°C. At the end of the incubation, shacked the 96 micro-well plates for 15 s. The optical density (OD) of the culture plate was read at a wavelength of 490 nm (reference absorbance at a wavelength of 630 nm) on an ELISA reader (Anthos 2020 spectrophotometer).

- **% cell survival:** $100 - \{(At - Ab) / (Ac - Ab)\} \times 100$

Where, At = absorbance of test, Ab = absorbance of blank

Ac = absorbance of control

- **% cell inhibition:** 100 – % cell survival

3.10. Statistical Package for the Social Sciences (SPSS)

SPSS is one of the most used programs for statistical analysis in social science. The program is used in many fields. Education researchers, market researchers, health researchers, survey companies, even the government, all use this program.

SPSS has a set of features which simplify programming. The program's datasets contain a table structure with rows and columns. The rows represent cases and the columns represent measurements like age, sex, etc. It has only 2 defined data types (text and numeric). SPSS Statistics 17.0.2 will help users in different fields to work together and obtain the best results for their companies.

These are some important features of SPSS 17.0.2:

- SPSS Missing Values add-on module (a feature that allows you to estimate data in case of missing files)
- Enhanced Syntax Editor: a features that creates, corrects, and test syntaxes fast and with a very small number of errors
- It can generate new interfaces, so that even beginners will consider the program easy to use

Objectives

To understand the analysis of variance models, *F* test for simultaneously comparing factors with respect to their means, the least-significant difference test: the ANOVA table.

ANOVA^b

	Model	Sum of Squares	*df*	Mean Square	F	Sig.
1	Regression	RSS	K-1	RSS/TSS		
	Residual	RSS	N*K-1	RSS/TSS	MSS/TSS	
	Total	TSS	N-I	SST+SSE		
	ERROR	ESS	N-K			

Table 3. ANOVA table

http://dx.doi.org/10.5772/61891

4. Results and discussion

4.1. Metal analysis

4.1.1. Metal analysis of soil

The elements that are present in the soil sample of the Malkapuram industrial polluted area and the less-polluted agency area Paderu of Visakha district in Andhra Pradesh were selected for study. There are 24 elements that were detected, namely, As, Ba, Co, Cr, Cu, Mo, Ni, Pb, Rb, Sr, V, Y, Zn, Zr, SiO_2, $A1_2O_3$, Fe_2O_3, MnO, MgO, CaO, Na_2O, K_2O, TiO_2, and P_2O_5 (Table 3). Among which nine are essentials elements (Fe, Co, Mg, Cu, Mo, V, Cr, Mn, and Ni). Mo is the heaviest and is relatively less abundant on the earth's crust. In our analysis of natural and polluted soils, Ni was not detected and Mo is in lower concentrations in natural sources and not detected in polluted soils. Cu is not detected in natural soils and is more abundant in polluted soils. Zn, Co, Cr, and V are more in polluted soils approximately four times. Fe and Mn are in oxide form with no significant increase in polluted soils.

Soil Elements	Natural Source	Polluted Source
As	5.35	6.2
Ba	519.4	857.5
Co	6.05	27.3
Cr	57.8	211
Cu	ND	33.6
Mo	5.2	ND
Ni	ND	ND
Pb	31.8	43
Rb	176.4	44.5
Sr	86.25	104.2
V	43.4	181.4
Y	49.7	25.7
Zn	71.65	338.8
Zr	216.25	177.3
SiO_2	84.4	53.6
Al_2O_3	8.2	6.38
Fe_2O_3	1.7	6.19
MnO	0.06	0.16
MgO	0.59	0.8
CaO	ND	3.26
Na_2O	1.1	1
K_2O	11.9	4.88
TiO_2	0.68	1.86
P_2O_5	0.1	1.79

Table 4. The concentrations of metal elements in the natural and polluted soils Testing of hypothesis for the data (*T* test):

All the representative metals (Na, K, Mg, P, and Ca) are in oxide form in soils and are found at higher concentrations in the soils of both natural and polluted sources. Si is one of the abundant elements on the earth's crust and has been found to be probably essential in one family of plants [40]. Si is present at higher ranges in both soils with not much significant variation. Analysis of five essential nonmetals (C, N, O, S, and Cl) was not included in the analysis. Al, Ti, and Zr are not essential, yet abundant in earth's crust and form extremely insoluble oxides. The presence of Al, Ti, and Zr show no significant variation in natural and polluted soils. As, Y, Sr, Rb, Pb, Ba, V, and Zr appear to be nonnutrient elements. They are neither included in the above essentiality list nor show significant variation in polluted and natural soils.

	Paired Differences					T	df	Sig. (2-tailed)
	Mean	Std. Deviation	Std. Error Mean	95% Confidence Interval of the Difference				
				Lower	Upper			
Natural source– - polluted source	6.039	108.491	24.259	86.814	14.736	1.486	19	.154

Table 5. Sample *T* test

The null hypothesis and alternative hypothesis with respect to natural and polluted soils can be stated as follows:

H_0: There is no significant difference between metals in polluted and natural soils

H_1: There is a significant difference between metals in polluted and natural soils

The *t*-statistic value is 1.486 and the significance is 0.154, which is more than 0.05, so the null hypotheses H_0 is not accepted. Hence, it is concluded that polluted soils showed higher concentrations than the natural soils.

4.1.2. (A) Comparison of metal analysis in natural and polluted sources

In a comparative study of these metals grown in polluted and natural sources, the concentration of 15 metals, namely, As Ba, Co, Cr, Cu, Pb, Sr, Zn, Al, Fe, Mn, Mg, Mo, Ti, and P are found to be higher in polluted soils than that of natural soils. This high concentration may be attributed to the release of elements from the surrounding industries of Malkapuram as the same are not found in control soil samples at higher concentrations. Our reasoning and results are in support that the abundant rock-forming elements are O, Al, Si, Fe, Na, K, Mg, and other than this major contribution to metal burden in soils, include discard-manufactured products as in scrap heaps, landfills (As, Cr, Cu, Pb, Mn, Zn), coal ashes (As, Cd, Pb, Mn, Mo, Ni, Se, V, and Zn), and agricultural wastes As, Cu, and Zn [41]. The United States Environmental Protection Agency (U.S. EPA) included 13 metals in their pollutants list: Ag, As, Be, Cd, Cr, Cu, Hg, Ni, Pb, Sb, Se, Ti, and Zn. Among the most important metals, Cd, Hg, Pb, Cr, and Zn are emitted from smelters and refineries. Cd, Se, and Hg are not analyzed in my study. The results are also consistent with the information given by several workers who accounted for the environmentally important metals As, Cd, Cr, Co, Hg, Pb, Mn, Ni, Se, and Zn and the less well-known but environmentally important elements Sb, Ba, Au, Mo, Ag, Th, Sn, Cu, U, and V [42].

In a comparative study of metals in polluted and natural soils, polluted soils showed higher concentrations than the natural soils and all heavy metals fall below the regulatory limits of the heavy metals applied to soils by the U.S. EPA [43] (Table 6).

Heavy Metals	Maximum Concentration in sludge mg/kg (ppm)	Concentration in natural soil	Concentration in polluted soil
As	75	5.35	6.2
Cd	85	ND	ND
Cr	3000	57.8	211
Cu	4300	ND	33.6
Pb	420	31.8	43
Hg	840	ND	ND
Mo	57	5.2	ND
Ni	75	ND	ND
Se	100	–	–
Zn	7500	71.65	338

ND = not detected.

Table 6. The heavy metal concentration of soils with regulatory limits. (Adapted from U.S. EPA 1993).

4.1.3. Analysis of metals in plant samples

A total of 26 elements (V, Cr, Mn, Ni, Co, Cu, Zn, As, Se, Rb, Sr, Mo, Ag, Cd, Sb, Ba, Ti, Pb, U, Na, Mg, Al, Si, K, Ca, and Fe) were estimated in the powdered medicinal plant samples of ten, each plant was grown under natural sources and plants thriving under polluted sources (Table 7).

Metal analysis was carried out in five medicinal plants, namely, *A. vasica (A.v), E. globulus (E.g), H. suaveolens (H.s), R. communis (R.c), and T. cordifolia (T.c)* from the Paderu region, which is considered to be a natural and less polluted area, and the same five plants from industrial polluted area of Malkapuram cluster. A total of 26 elements (V, Cr, Mn, Ni, Co, Cu, Zn, As, Se, Rb, Sr, Mo, Ag, Cd, Sb, Ba, Ti, Pb, U, Na, Mg, Al, Si, K, Ca, and Fe) were estimated in the 10 powdered medicinal plant samples, each of the plants were grown under natural sources and thriving under polluted sources. Among these, the role played by 15 elements (Na, Mg, Al, Si, K, Ca, V, Cr, Mn, Fe, Co, Ni, Cu, Zn, and Mo) as macro- and micronutrients to support the growth and development of the plants is established [44]. As, Se, Rb, Sr, Ag, Cd, Sb, Ba, Ti, Pb, and U are nonessential nutrients.

Ele	*A. vasica* (N)	*A. vasica* (P)	*E. globulus* (N)	*E. globulus* (P)	*H. suaveolens* (N)	*H. suaveolens* (P)	*R. communis* (N)	*R. communis* (P)	*T. cordifolia* (N)	*T. cordifolia* (P)
Fe	0.98796	1.77412	0.68672	1.01536	0.89097	4.2936	0.77276	2.1658	1.38922	0.63875
Co	0.00244	0.00192	0.00948	0.00084	0.00495	0.00474	0.00153	0.0019	0.00237	0.00072
Zn	0.67237	0.57145	0.55601	0.66609	0.38132	0.8085	0.46781	0.6722	0.68254	0.59659
Cu	0.08278	0.08773	0.06837	0.04879	0.09411	0.12817	0.06431	0.0916	0.14323	0.07426
Mo	0.00576	0.02651	0.02532	0.0092	0.00256	0.00383	0.113	0.0353	0.00193	0.00257
V	0.00335	0.00458	0.00299	0.00472	0.00333	0.01382	0.00338	0.0066	0.00693	0.00293
Cr	0.08009	0.09044	0.08066	0.0803	0.08188	0.10096	0.07854	0.0866	0.08381	0.0847
Mn	0.2382	0.20703	4.98842	0.64406	0.60595	0.64673	0.38399	0.4353	0.43473	0.1411
Ni	0.2768	0.03153	0.04767	0.03006	0.02322	0.03344	0.02246	0.0271	0.03843	0.01687
The concentration of essential trace elements (in ppm) in both treated and control plants										
Na	4.095	5.42096	9.95389	25.6549	4.33451	11.0924	4.96097	7.0729	5.77424	10.1774
K	230.648	223.862	67.4462	84.3537	181.501	122.72	234.129	162.33	223.08	247.791
Mg	32.274	64.4634	12.3217	9.15043	27.363	33.8241	23.8091	33.627	15.4185	12.7332
Ca	208.215	261.432	82.4995	52.9004	133.748	144.43	134.994	190.48	85.0588	55.856
The concentration of representative elements (in ppm) in treated and control plants										
Al	0.69115	0.7559	0.56936	0.64118	0.96181	1.87821	0.74413	1.2689	1.46868	0.62012
TI	0.00026	0.00023	0.00013	0.00021	0.00008	0.00026	0.00008	0.0002	0.0001	0.0007
The concentration of nonessential trace elements (in ppm) in both treated and control plants										
Si	2.08043	2.42939	2.23198	2.20235	2.28226	1.9138	2.24237	2.5118	1.86681	2.36288
As	0.0012	0.00205	0.00163	0.00173	0.00122	0.00569	0.00127	0.0031	0.00189	0.0012
Se	0.15301	0.16083	0.17753	0.15543	0.14497	0.16998	0.14665	0.1579	0.14961	0.16122
Rb	0.14468	0.0914	0.15147	0.02595	0.23845	0.09003	0.16182	0.0855	0.1105	0.23519
Sr	0.48	0.77235	0.21404	0.20187	0.58336	0.3376	0.38586	0.4858	0.26037	0.1645
Ag	0.00047	0.00046	0.00061	0.00035	0.00051	0.00059	0.00064	0.0006	0.00046	0.00046
Cd	0.00331	0.00159	0.00134	0.0029	0.00181	0.00259	0.00101	0.002	0.00128	0.0012
Sb	0.00016	0.00025	0.00023	0.00026	0.00021	0.00057	0.00016	0.0004	0.00023	0.00034
Ba	0.30367	0.16086	0.28909	0.2944	1.28744	0.12151	0.18919	0.1079	0.24005	0.06183
Pb	0.02018	0.02472	0.01214	0.03141	0.02817	0.03618	0.0162	0.0259	0.192	0.02445
U	0.00026	0.00049	0.00022	0.00092	0.00025	0.00122	0.00024	0.0007	0.00034	0.00042
The concentration of toxic, heavy metals (in ppm) in treated and control plants										
N = natural P = polled										

Table 7. The concentration of metals (in ppm) in treated and control plants

http://dx.doi.org/10.5772/61891

The results supported the information given by Craig Dick (2008), who said that there are actually 20 mineral elements necessary or beneficial for plant growth. Carbon (C), hydrogen (H), and oxygen (O) are supplied by air and water.

The six macronutrients, nitrogen (N), phosphorus (P), potassium (K), calcium (Ca), magnesium (Mg), and sulfur (S) are required by plants in large amounts. The rest of the elements are required in trace amounts (micronutrients). Essential trace elements include boron (B), chlorine (Cl), copper (Cu), iron (Fe), manganese (Mn), sodium (Na), zinc (Zn), molybdenum (Mo), and nickel (Ni). Beneficial mineral elements include silicon (Si) and cobalt (Co). The beneficial elements have not been deemed essential for all plants but may be essential for some. The distinction between beneficial and essential is often difficult in the case of some trace elements.

The data in Table 7 indicates the uptake of elements (macro, trace, and heavy elements) by the various medicinal plants grown in natural and polluted areas and their comparative analysis is drawn. All the plants grown in polluted areas having more than 12 elements in higher concentration than the natural ones. The descending order in the number of metals found are 21, 18, 15, 13, and 12, respectively, in *R. communis (R.c), H. suaveolens (H.s), A. vasica (A.v), E. globulus (E.g)*, and *T. cordifolia (T.c)*. The concentration of metals in natural conditions is less than in polluted conditions. This is because heavy metal pollution can arise from many sources, or more precisely, the activities are carried out in seven industries that are surrounding my area of study. Therefore, the sources of these metals in soils and plants are the industries. There are many correlations observed in the elemental content of both natural and polluted conditions. The metals, even though they are present in soil, the uptake by plants are seemingly less.

	Test value = 0					
	T	*df*	Sig. (2-tailed)	Mean Difference	95% Confidence Interval of the Difference	
					Lower	Upper
A.V (N)	1.585	25	.125	18.5177127	−5.541360	42.576786
A.V(P)	1.659	25	.110	21.62977654	−5.2224022	48.4819552
E.G(N)	1.757	25	.091	7.0129500	−1.208756	15.234656
E.G(P)	1.797	25	.084	6.85068500	−0.9992846	14.7006546
H.S(N)	1.608	25	.120	13.63712846	−3.8335830	31.1078399
H.S(P)	1.736	25	.095	12.4099431	−2.311420	27.131306
R.C(N)	1.525	25	.140	15.52655654	−5.4409577	36.4940708
R.C(P)	1.641	25	.113	15.4493462	−3.942021	34.840713
T.C(N)	1.434	25	.164	12.9387327	−5.645728	31.523193
T.C(P)	1.322	25	.198	12.7596385	−7.119869	32.639146

Table 8. Sample *T* test

Testing of hypothesis for the data (*T*-test)

The *t*-statistic values for different metals are in the above table and significance values are greater than 0.05. So, null hypotheses H_0 is not accepted. Hence, it is concluded that polluted soils showed higher concentrations than the natural soils.

In all the plants that have been studied for metal uptake, six elements, namely, Na, Mg, Al, Si, K, and Ca, are found in high concentrations in both control and polluted plants, ranging from 4 to 354 ppm, whereas Fe shows in *Tinospora*, respectively, ranging between 001 and 5.48 ppm, which is enumerated in Table 7, whereas all other 19 elements fall below 1 ppm in all plants. In addition, this metal concentration is high in plants grown in polluted areas than from the natural areas.

From the study, it was revealed that all the metals accumulated to a greater or lesser extent by all plant species studied. The plants showed a large number of elements and were rich in Na, Mg, Ca, K, Fe, Al, and Si, which are earth's crust elements and the same were found to be abundant in earth's crust also. There is a lot of correlation observed in the elemental content of both soils and plants studied in the natural and polluted conditions.

The higher concentrations of 7 metals (Na, Mg, Al, Si, K, Ca, and Fe) are seen in polluted plants, except for Na, which is highest in the natural condition.

Na ranges between 4.095 and 26.655 ppm, and the highest concentration is seen in *E. globulus* (polluted) having 26.655 ppm. Mg ranges between 9.150 and 64.463 ppm and the highest concentration is seen in *A. vasica* (polluted) having 64.463 ppm. Al ranges between 0.569 and 1.878 ppm and the highest concentration is seen in *H. suaveolens* (polluted) having 1.878 ppm. Si ranges between 1.867 and 2.512 ppm and the highest concentration is seen in *R. communis* (polluted) having 2.513 ppm. K ranges between 67.446 and 247.791 ppm and the highest concentration is seen in *T. cordifolia* (polluted) having 247.791 ppm. Ca ranges between 52.900 and 261.432 ppm and the highest concentration is seen in *A. vasica* (polluted) having 261.432 ppm. Fe ranges between 0.1749 and 4.988 ppm and the highest concentration is seen in *E. globulus* (natural) having 5.484 ppm (Figs. 1–5).

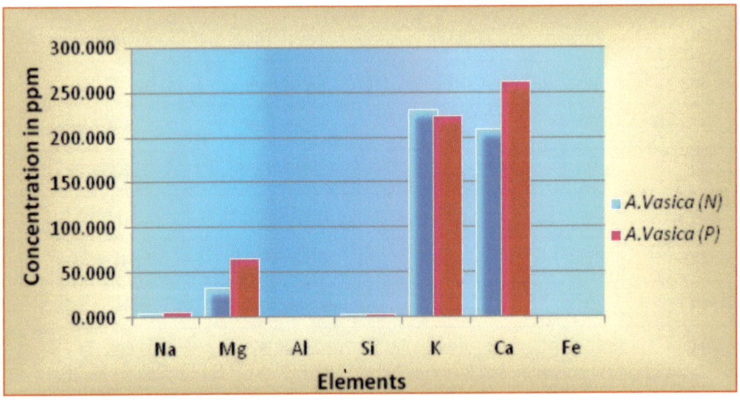

Figure 1. Metals with higher concentration in *A. vasica* (AV) Polluted (P) natural (N).

http://dx.doi.org/10.5772/61891

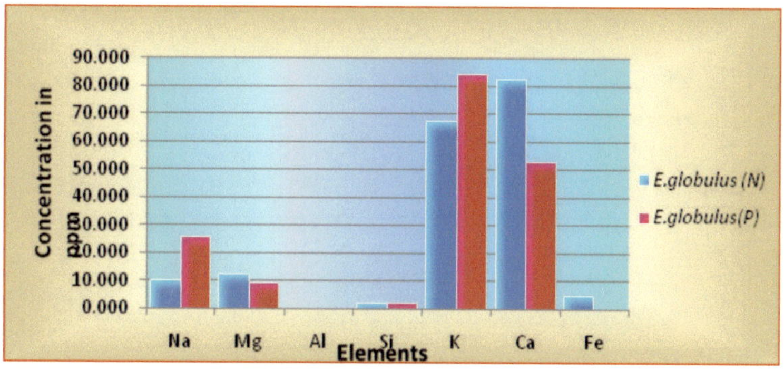

Figure 2. Metals with higher concentration in *E. globulus* (EG) polluted (P) natural (N).

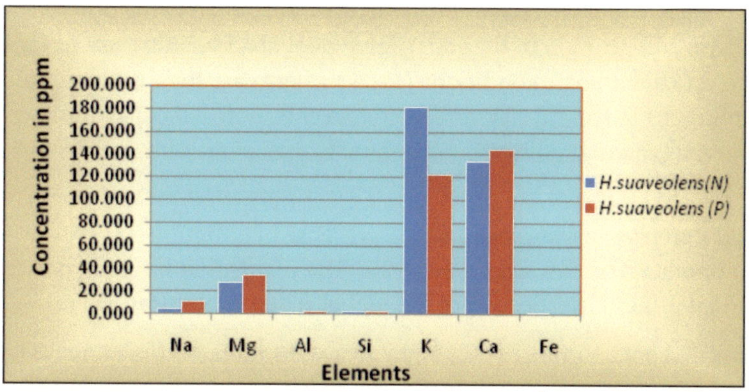

Figure 3. Metals with higher concentration in *H. suaveolens* (HS) polluted (P) natural (N).

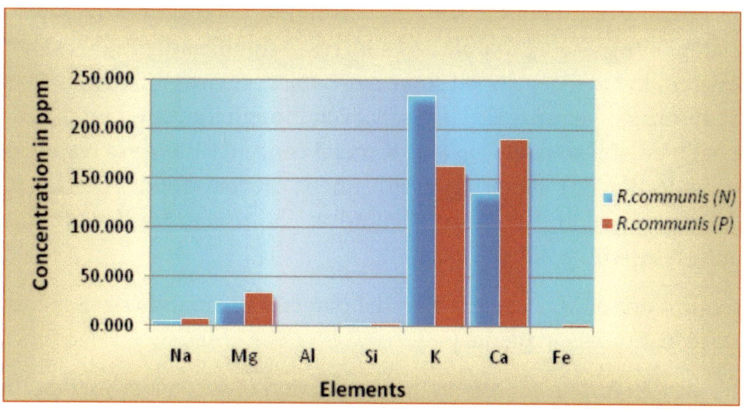

Figure 4. Metals with higher concentration in *R. communis* (RC) polluted (P) natural (N).

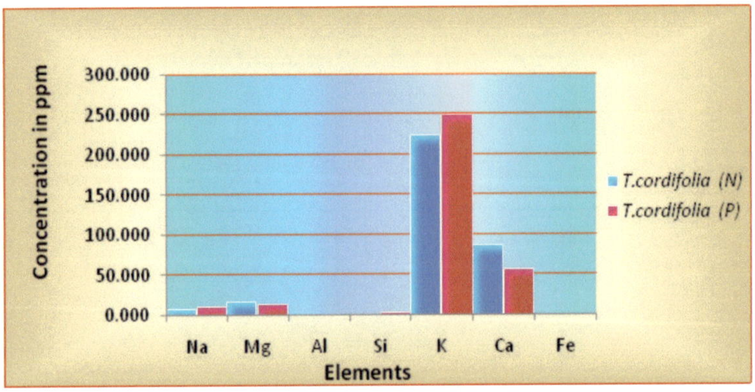

Figure 5. Metals with higher concentration in *T. cordifolia* (TC) polluted (P) natural (N).

The variations in elemental concentration are mainly attributed to the differences in botanical structure, mineral composition of the soil, preferential absorbability, use of fertilizers, irrigation of water, and climatologic conditions [45]. Furthermore, the difference in sampling and presence of pollution sources can also effect the concentration of metals from species to species. The plants that are grown in polluted areas show luxuriant growth irrespective of the higher metal concentration.

Furthermore, differences in sampling and the presence of pollution sources can also affect the concentration of metals from species to species. The plants that are grown in polluted areas showed luxuriant growth irrespective of the higher metal concentration.

Of the elements that are accumulated in higher concentration, Na (in all plants) and Co and Si (in two plants) are beneficial elements. In the above plants showing luxuriant growth in polluted sources, the beneficial elements could be compensating for the toxic effects of other elements or replacing the mineral nutrients in some other less specific function such as maintenance of osmotic pressure. Also, it is surprising to know that the percentage of Na in the soils of both natural and polluted sources was found to be almost the same., and yet, the Na uptake by all plants growing in polluted sources is significantly higher. The reason could be that the plants could have developed some mechanism such as ion flux, which may prevent the plant from absorbing heavy toxic elements even though they are found in higher concentration in the polluted soil sources. Na and K metal concentrations are responsible for maintaining normal hydration and osmotic pressure and K concentration is needed for cell growth and function. Thus, the high content of K could be the reason for the luxuriant growth of medicinal plants in heavily polluted areas.

The high concentrations of Mg, Ca, and K in the plants show that these elements are the most abundant metal constituents in plants [46].

Trace elements play an important role in the production of secondary metabolites, which are responsible for the pharmacological actions of medicinal plants [47]. Furthermore, it is aimed to study the concentration of these metals that are listed at higher level in the selected medicinal plants and later to intensify the study on their biological effects. In general, it is observed in my study that even though the concentration of metal elements is high in soil, the uptake of metals by plants is seemingly less.

4.1.4. (a) Heavy metals and medicinal plants

The heavy metal concentration with permissible limits [56] FAO/WHO 1984: In all 5 plants studied out of 11 heavy metals detected, namely, Zn, As, Co, Cu, Cd, Ti, Pb, Ni, Mn, Fe, and Cr. More than 9 metals are in high concentration in plants grown in polluted than in plants grown in natural condition (Table 9). All plants grown in natural and polluted areas have metal concentrations that are below the permissible limits of the FAO/WHO (1984). Zn and Pb concentrations in all plants grown in polluted areas are high when compared to plants grown in natural areas [48].

Elements	FAO/WHO limits	*A. vasica* (N)	*A. vasica* (P)	*E. globulus* (N)	*E. globulus* (P)	*H. suaveolens* (N)	*H. suaveolens* (P)	*R. communis* (N)	*R. communis* (P)	*T. cordifolia* (N)	*T. cordifolia* (P)
Zn	27.4	0.67237	0.55601	0.38132	0.46781	0.68254	0.57145	0.66609	0.8085	0.67223	0.59659
As	1	0.0012	0.00163	0.00122	0.00127	0.00189	0.00205	0.00173	0.00569	0.00306	0.0012
Co	0.48	0.00244	0.00948	0.00495	0.00153	0.00237	0.00192	0.00084	0.00474	0.00185	0.00072
Cu	3	0.08278	0.06837	0.09411	0.06431	0.14323	0.08773	0.04879	0.12817	0.09162	0.07426
Cd	0.21	0.00331	0.00134	0.00181	0.00101	0.00128	0.00159	0.0029	0.00259	0.00203	0.0012
TI		0.00026	0.00013	0.00008	0.00008	0.0001	0.00023	0.00021	0.00026	0.00017	0.0007
Pb	0.43	0.02018	0.01214	0.02817	0.0162	0.192	0.02472	0.03141	0.03618	0.02588	0.02445
Ni	1.63	0.2768	0.04767	0.02322	0.02246	0.03843	0.03153	0.03006	0.03344	0.02708	0.01687
Mn	2.001	0.2382	4.98842	0.60595	0.38399	0.43473	0.20703	0.64406	0.64673	0.43534	0.1411
Fe	20	0.98796	0.68672	0.89097	0.77276	1.38922	1.77412	1.01536	4.2936	2.16584	0.63875
Cr	0.02	0.08009	0.08066	0.08188	0.07854	0.08381	0.09044	0.0803	0.10096	0.08655	0.0847

Table 9. Heavy metal concentration in plants with permissible limits of FAO/WHO 1984 (ppm)

The *t*-statistic value for different metals in Table 10 are greater than 0.05. So, null hypotheses H_0 is not accepted, i.e., in all the 5 plants studied, out of 11 heavy metals detected, namely, Zn, As, Co, Cu, Cd, Ti, Pb, Ni, Mn, Fe, and Cr. More than 9 metals are in high concentration in plants grown in polluted conditions than natural conditions.

Copper (Cu): The copper concentrations in all polluted plants are high, ranging between 0.04879 and 0.12817 than the unpolluted plants, which range between 0.06431 and 0.1472. The permissible limits of FAO/WHO for copper (Cu) is 3 ppm. Copper is an essential enzymatic element for normal plant growth and development but can be toxic at excessive levels. Phytotoxicity can occur if its concentration in plants is higher than 20 mg/kg DW (dry weight).

	Paired Differences					*T*	*df*	Sig. (2-tailed)
	Mean	Std. Deviation	Std. Error Mean	95% Confidence Interval of the Difference				
				Lower	Upper			
FAO/WHO - A.V(N)	5.380567	9.435203	2.983673	−1.368971016	1.213010502E1	1.803	9	.105
FAO/WHOE.G(N)	4.971856	9.819888	3.105321	−2.052869174	1.199658117E1	1.601	9	.144
FAO/WHO - H.S(N)	5.405740	9.529765	3.013576	−1.411443352	1.222292335E1	1.794	9	.106
FAO/WHO - R.C(N)	5.436112	9.514774	3.008835	−1.370347592	1.224257159E1	1.807	9	.104
FAO/WHO - T.C(N)	5.320150	9.378580	2.965767	−1.388882144	1.202918214E1	1.794	9	.106
FAO/WHO - A.V(P)	5.337842	9.325711	2.949048	−1.333370270	1.200905427E1	1.810	9	.104
FAO/WHO - E.G(P)	5.364946	9.438893	2.984840	−1.387231321	1.211712332E1	1.797	9	.106
FAO/WHO - H.S(P)	5.011040	8.924020	2.822023	−1.372819819	1.139489982E1	1.776	9	.110
FAO/WHO - R.C(P)	5.265952	9.249872	2.925066	−1.351008190	1.188291219E1	1.800	9	.105
FAO/WHO - T.C(P)	5.459116	9.494573	3.002447	−1.332892374	1.225112437E1	1.818	9	.102

Table 10. Sample *T* test

The critical concentration for copper in plants is 20–100 mg/kg [49]. As with other heavy metals, some species can tolerate very high amounts of copper [50].

Cadmium (Cd): The cadmium concentrations in all polluted plants are high, ranging between 0.001 and 0.0029 compared with that of unpolluted plants, which range between 0.00101 and 0.0033. The permissible limit of FAO/WHO for cadmium (Cd) is 0.21 ppm. Cadmium is a toxic metal having functions neither in human body nor in animals or plants [51].

Tin (Ti): The tin concentration in all polluted plants is high, ranging from 0.0001 to 0.0007 compared with that of unpolluted plants, which range between 0.00008 and 0.0026. The permissible limit of FAO/WHO for tin is (TI) not set.

Lead (Pb): The concentration of lead in all the plants grown in polluted areas is higher than the natural conditions. The concentration of lead in both types falls below the permissible limits of FAO/WHO for lead (Pb), which is 0.43 ppm. The concentration of lead in all plants grown in polluted areas ranges from 0.0244 to 0.03618, and the concentration of lead in all plants grown in natural conditions is 0.0121–0.2821. Lead is regarded as very hazardous for plants and humans [52]. Obviously, the high lead concentration in the aerial parts of plants from polluted areas is due to the lead coming from the emission of vehicles as well as its presence in the soils polluted with wastes from different operations [53].

Nickel (Ni): The nickel concentrations in all polluted plants are high, ranging between 0.0168 and 0.0384 compared with that of unpolluted plants, which range between 0.022 and 0.2744. The permissible limit of FAO/WHO for nickel (Ni) is 1.63 ppm. Nickel is an abundant element;

it is required in minute quantities for the body as it is mostly present in the pancreas and hence plays an important role in the production of insulin. Its deficiency results in a disorder of the liver [54].

Manganese (Mn): The manganese concentration in all polluted plants ranges between 0.141 and 0.64673 compared with that of unpolluted plants, which range between 0.238 and 4.9884. The permissible limit of FAO/WHO for manganese (Mn) is 2.001 ppm.

Manganese is also an essential element for plant and animal growth. Its uptake is controlled metabolically. Soils derive manganese from the parent material and its contents in rocks is higher than the concentration of other micronutrients apart from iron [55]. The main sources of manganese in the soil are fertilizers, sewage sludge, and ferrous smelters.

Iron (Fe): The iron concentrations in all polluted plants are high, ranging between 0.6387 and 4.2936, whereas that of the unpolluted plants range between 0.6867 and 1.3892. The permissible limit of FAO/WHO for iron (Fe) is 20 ppm.

Iron is very essential for plants and animals. Its deficiency in plants produces chlorosis disease; however, high concentrations also affect plant growth. The plant samples were collected from polluted areas and, in general, the concentrations of iron in polluted areas are higher.

Chromium (Cr): The chromium concentrations in all polluted plants are high, ranging between 0.0803 and 0.10096, whereas that of the unpolluted plants range between 0.07854 and 0.08381. The permissible limit of FAO/WHO for chromium (Cr) is 0.2 ppm.

Chromium is one of known environmental toxic pollutants in the world. The main sources of chromium contamination are tanneries, steel industries, sewage sludge application, and fly ash [56].

Pb, Cd, and Fe also accumulated more in plants growing in polluted sources. Higher concentrations of Pb and Cd in plants grown in polluted sources might reflect the concentration of these commonly encountered metals in polluted soils, which are being continuously released from the surrounding industries such as Coromandel Fertilizers, Hindustan Petroleum Corporation Limited, Hindustan Shipyard, steel plants, etc. Chelate-assisted phytoextraction has been developed because plants do not naturally accumulate important toxic elements, e.g., Pb, Cd, and As, that would be significant in remediation: continuous phytoextraction of metals relies on the properties of plant that lead to accumulation in aerial plant tissues [57].

Positively, the concentration of heavy metals in my study falls below the permissible limits and thus do not interrupt any regular functions of the plant and this could be the reason why plants grown in polluted areas have normal and luxuriant growth.

The heavy metal concentrations in my results were justified by the works of Yadav (2010), where plants experience oxidative stress upon exposure to heavy metals that leads to cellular damage and disturbance of cellular ionic homeostasis. To minimize the detrimental effects of heavy metal exposure and their accumulation, plants have evolved detoxification mechanisms mainly based on chelation and subcellular compartmentalization. These reasons also could support why the concentration of heavy metals did not affect the growth of plants in the polluted areas of my study [58].

4.2. Phytochemical analysis

The five plants that have luxuriant growth have been selected for further study after metal analysis. The phytochemical characteristics of five medicinal plants grown in polluted and natural conditions were tested. The results revealed the presence of medically active compounds in methanolic extracts (Table 11). Almost all plants showed the presence of phytochemicals, namely, terpenoids, flavonoids, phenols, and alkaloids either in polluted or in control extracts of methanolic solvent. Hexane and chlorofoam showed no presence of phytochemicals.

Sample	Terpenoid	Flavonoids	Phenols	Saponins	Alkaloids
A. vasica Nees, (N)	+	+	+	–	+
A. vasica Nees (P)	–	–	–	–	+
E. globulus (Labille) (N)	+	+	+	–	–
E. globulus (Labille) (P)	+	+	+	–	+
H. suaveolens,(L.) Poit. (N)	+	+	+	–	+
H. suaveolens,(L.) Poit. (P))	–	+	+	–	+
R. communis Linn. (N)	+	+	–	–	–
R. communis Linn. (P)	+	+	+	–	–
T. cordifolia, Miers (N)	+	–	+	–	–
T. cordifolia, Miers (P)	+	+	-	-	+

Table 11. Preliminary phytochemical analyses of selected medicinal plants from natural and polluted sources

In addition, my work is supported by the results of Arvind Kumar et al. (2014), where methanolic extracts showed the presence of a large number of phytochemicals [59]. The results showed the concentration of phenols, flavonoids, and alkaloids in methanolic extracts. Flavonoids are not found in hexane and chloroform extracts [60]. The methanolic extract showed greater inhibition against *Pseudomonas* and *B. subtilis*. According to the results of Venkataswamy [61], the methanolic extracts showed the presence of flavonoids and triterpenoids. The presence of tannins and saponins are in contrast to my results. Except in *A. vasica* and *H. squaveolens*, all other three plants, namely, *Eucalyptus*, *Ricinus*, and *Tinospora* from polluted areas showed more phytochemicals than the plants grown in natural conditions. Flavonoids and phenols are seen in polluted plants of *Eucalyptus*, *Ricinus*, and *Hyptis* whereas alkaloids are seen in *Adhotoda* and *Hyptis* of both control and polluted plants.

4.2.1. Preliminary phytochemical analysis

The preliminary phytochemical analysis of plants showed that flavonoids, phenols, terpenoids, and alkaloids are seen in plants *A. vasika* and *H. suaveolens* that are grown in natural conditions and in *E. globulus* that is grown in polluted conditions.

http://dx.doi.org/10.5772/61891

The results obtained in this study thus suggest that the identified phytochemical compounds may be bioactive constituents and that these plants are proving to be an increasing valuable reservoir of bioactive compounds of substantial medicinal merit. The results are at par with the results of Daniel and Daniang (2011), where many phytochemicals found in plants are either the products of plant metabolism or synthesized for defense purposes [62].

A. vasica has all four phytochemicals in natural condition, only alkaloids in *A. vasica* were polluted. In *Eucalyptus*, except for alkaloids, all three flavonoids, phenols, and terpenoids are found in both plants. But alkaloids present only in polluted plants, this is confirmed where the crude extract of medicinal plant studied was found to contain one or more of the following phytochemical compounds flavonoids, phenols, terpenoids, alkaloids, and volatile oils [63]. Other investigators have reported the presence of these components in members of the family Myrtaceae to which the plant used in the present study belongs. The inhibitory effects of this medicinal plant on the microorganisms may therefore be due to the presence of the above phytochemical components [64].

In *Hyptis* flavonoids, phenols, and alkaloids are found in both types of plants. Terpenoids are present only in plants in the natural condition. *Ricinus* (natural) has only terpenoids and flavonoids but *Ricinus* (polluted) has terpenoids, flavonoids, and phenols. *T. cordifolia* (natural) has only terpenoids and phenols and *T. cordifolia* (polluted) has terpenoids, flavonoids, and alkaloids. The presence of phenols in all five plants except in *A. vasica* (polluted), *R. communis* (natural), *T. cordifolia* (polluted) may help these plants to be very effective in their usage as a herbal medicine.

As the previous studies explained that phenolic compounds are one of the largest and most ubiquitous groups of plant metabolites [59]. They possess biological properties such as antiapoptosis, antiaging, anticarcinogen, anti-inflammation, antiatherosclerosis, cardiovascular protection, and improvement of endothelial function as well as inhibition of angiogenesis and cell proliferation activities [65].

The flavonoid contents of the plants in my study are consistent with the results of Okwu, as flavonoids are hydroxylated phenolic substances known to be synthesized by plants in response to microbial infection and they have been found to have antimicrobial substances against a wide array of microorganisms in vitro [66].

The results also showed the presence of alkaloids in *A. vasica* (natural), *A. vasica* (polluted), *E. globulus* (polluted), *H. suoveolens* (natural), *H. suoveolens* (polluted), and in *T. cordifolia* (polluted). Alkaloids have been associated with medicinal uses for centuries and one of their common biological properties is their cytotoxicity [67, 68]. Several workers have reported the analgesic, antispasmodic, and antibacterial properties of alkaloids.

The investigations have opened up the possibilities of the use of these plants in drug development for human consumption possibly for the treatment of gastrointestinal, urinary tract, wound infections, and typhoid fever. Preliminary phytochemical analysis revealed the presence of phenols, terpenoids alkaloids, and flavonoids. It is not surprising that there are differences in the antibacterial effects of plant groups due to phytochemicals properties and different among species.

4.2.2. Quantitative analysis of phenols and flavonoids

The amount of total phenols was determined with the Folin–Ciocalteu reagent. Galic acid was used as a standard compound and the total phenols were expressed as μg/mg gallic acid equivalent using the standard curve equation: $y = 0.0061x + 0.0396$, $R^2 = 0.9991$, where y is absorbance at 760 nm and x is total phenolic content in the different extracts expressed in mg/g. Phenolic compounds are a class of antioxidant agents which act as free radical terminators [69].

Except for *A. vasica*, all four plants *E. globulus* (polluted): 279.4, *H. suoveolens* (polluted): 298, *R. communis* (polluted): 80.36, and *T. cordifolia* (polluted): 283.6 showed high concentrations of phenols compared with controls (Fig. 6). Interestingly, *Adhatoda* shows lower concentrations than controls. The highest concentration is seen in *H. suoveolens* (polluted) with 298 μg/mg. The next highest was *E. globulus* (polluted) at 279.4 μg/mg.

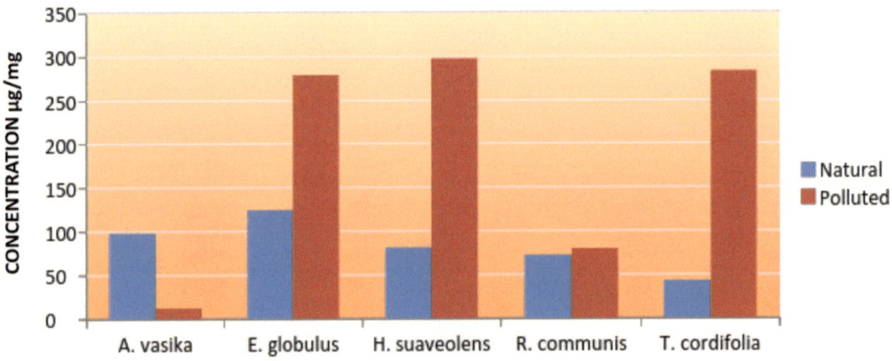

Figure 6. Total phenol content in plants grown in natural and polluted areas.

	Test Value = 0					
	t	*df*	Sig. (2-tailed)	Mean Difference	95% Confidence Interval of the Difference	
					Lower	Upper
GAE (μg/mg dry mass for methanol)	4.038	9	.003	1.373582	60.4171333	214.2988667

Table 12. One-sample test

Testing of hypothesis for the data (*T*-test)

The *t*-statistic value is 4.038, that is, more than 0.05. So, the null hypotheses H_0 is not accepted. Hence, it is concluded that except for *A. vasica*, all other four plants *E. globulus, H. suoveolens, R. communis*, and *T. cordifolia* showed high concentrations of phenols than controls.

http://dx.doi.org/10.5772/61891

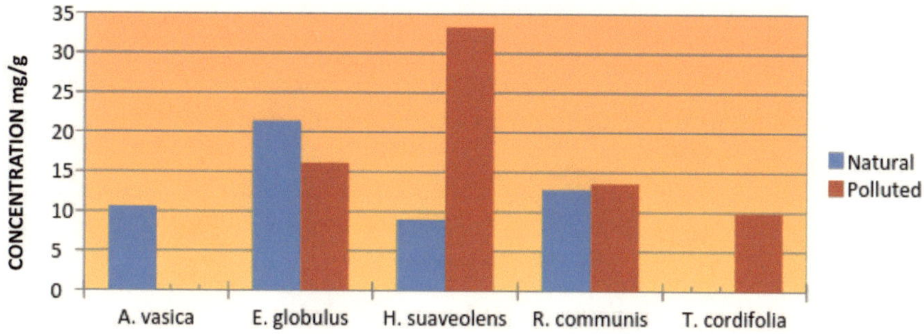

Figure 7. Total flavonoid content in plants grown in natural and polluted areas.

Estimation of flavonoid content using Swain and Hillis method (1959) used by Zachariah et al. (2012) employed in my work to estimate flavonoids [70]. In our results, high concentrations of flavonoids were found in *H. suoveolens* (polluted): 33.1 mg/g, *R. communis* (polluted): 13.6 mg/g, and *T. cordifolia* (polluted) in comparison with their natural varieties that have 19 mg/g, 12.8 mg/g, and 0 concentrations, respectively (Table 16). Three out of five plants from polluted areas showed high flavonoid contents and the remaining two showed low concentrations than the plants grown in natural conditions. The highest concentration is observed in *H. suoveolens* (polluted) is 33.1 mg/g (Figure 7).

		Paired Differences					*T*	*df*	Sig. (2-tailed)
		Mean	Std. Deviation	Std. Error Mean	95% Confidence Interval of the Difference				
					Lower	Upper			
Pair 1	Conc. of Flavonoids mg/g of dried extract nol	1.3191	4.212	1.59221	−1.7087	−9.2955	4.285	6	.000

Table 13. Paired samples test

The value of the *t*-statistic calculated is 4.285. The values of the *T*-statistic are greater than 0.05. So the null hypotheses H_0 is not accepted, i.e., that out of three plants from polluted areas showed high flavonoid content and the remaining two showed lower concentrations than plants grown in natural conditions. Therefore, polluted has high concentration.

4.2.3. The relationship between heavy metal concentration and phytochemicals

Table 14 shows the 11 heavy metals detected and 4 out of 5 plants, *E. globulus, H. sauveolens, R. communis,* and *T. cordifolia* except for *A. vasica,* have heavy metal concentrations that are higher in polluted plants than in controls. Interestingly, the same four plants showed high numbers of phytochemicals and quantity of phenols. But only two plants (*R. communis* and *T.*

cordifolia) showed high quantities of flavonoids. This indicated that there is a positive correlation existing between heavy metal concentration and phytochemical concentrations. The works of Milan and Stankovic, where birches grown in polluted substance showed higher total phenols than birches grown in unpolluted areas, support my present work.

Plants		Heavy Metal Concentration (PPM)											Total Phenolic (μg/mg)	Total Flavonoids (mg/g)
		As	Cd	Cr	Cu	Pb	Co	Ni	Zn	Mn	Fe	Ti		
A. vasica Nees	N	0.0012	0.00331	0.08009	0.08278	0.02018	0.00244	0.2768	0.67237	0.2382	0.98796	0.00026	98.26	10.6
	P	0.00205	0.00159	0.09044	0.08773	0.02472	0.00192	0.03153	0.57145	0.20703	1.77412	0.00023	12.68	ND
E. globulus	N	0.00163	0.00134	0.08066	0.06837	0.01214	0.00948	0.04767	0.55601	4.98842	0.68672	0.00013	124.42	21.4
	P	0.00173	0.0029	0.0803	0.04879	0.03141	0.00084	0.03006	0.66609	0.64406	1.01536	0.00021	279.4	16.1
H. suaveolens	N	0.00122	0.00181	0.08188	0.09411	0.02817	0.00495	0.02322	0.38132	0.60595	0.89097	0.00008	81.5	9.00
	P	0.00569	0.00259	0.10096	0.12817	0.03618	0.00474	0.03344	0.8085	0.64673	4.2936	0.00026	298.4	33.3
R. communis	N	0.00127	0.00101	0.07854	0.06431	0.0162	0.00153	0.02246	0.46781	0.38399	0.77276	0.00008	72.5	12.8
	P	0.00306	0.00203	0.08655	0.09162	0.02588	0.00185	0.02708	0.67223	0.43534	2.16584	0.00017	80.34	13.6
T. cordifolia	N	0.00189	0.00128	0.08381	0.14323	0.192	0.14323	0.03843	0.68254	0.43473	1.38922	0.0001	42.86	ND
	P	0.0012	0.0012	0.0847	0.07426	0.02445	0.07426	0.01687	0.59659	0.1411	0.63875	0.0007	283.6	9.9

Table 14. The effect of metal concentration on the total phenols and flavonoids content

4.3. Antimicrobial activity

The hexane, chloroform, and methanol extracts of five plants, namely, *A. vasica,* Nees, *H. suaveolens,* (L.) Poit., *E. globulus,* Labill. *R. communis* Linn., and *T. cordifolia,* Meirs grown in both industrial polluted and natural areas were subjected to antimicrobial activity by using the well diffusion method. Table 2 shows the pathogens used, morphology, and the diseases they cause. All five plants in the study were treated against 8 pathogens (Table 2): *S. aureus, C. albicans, B. subtilis, Enterococcus, Shigella, Klebsiella, B. cereus,* and *E. coli.* Among the Gram-negative bacteria are *K. pneumonia, Shigella,* and *E. coli,* whereas the Gram-positive bacteria are *S. aureus, B. subtilis, B. cereus,* and *E. faecalis. C. albicans* is a fungus.

The overall results showed that all the plant extracts have antimicrobial activity against all Gram-positive bacteria, namely, *S. aureus, B. subtilis, B. cereus,* and *Enterococcus,* and the zone of inhibition between 5 and 20 mm is observed. These plant extracts have not shown any activity or insignificant activity against Gram-negative bacteria *Klebsiella, Shigella,* and *E. coli.* The zone of inhibition (ZOI) was analyzed in all the plants and among the three solvent extracts, the methanolic extract showed zones of inhibition better than the hexane and chloroform solvents, where they showed minimum or no zone of inhibition. The methanol extracts of all plants showed ZOI against all pathogens except *Shigella, Klebsiella,* and *E. coli* (Plates 4-6).

Methanolic extracts of *A. vasica* (natural) showed antimicrobial activity against all pathogens except *Shigella. A. vasica* (polluted) showed antimicrobial activity against *S. aureus, B. subtilis, B. cereus, C. albicans,* and *E. coli* (10 mm) only in methanol extracts. Methanolic extracts of *A. vasica* showed ZOI to all the pathogens varying between 7 and 12 mm except for *Enterococcus* and *Klebsiella*. The plants grown in natural areas has more ZOI (13 mm) against *C. albicans* when compared with the plants grown in industrial polluted areas. The least was 7 mm.

Among all five plant extracts, the extract of *E. globulus* (natural) and *E. globulus* (polluted) showed antimicrobial activity against all pathogens except *Klebsiella* and *E. coli*. The highest zone of inhibition was 20 mm against *B. cereus* in *E. globulus* (natural) and 18 mm in *E. globulus* (polluted). All the pathogens except *Klebsiella* and *E. coli* were susceptible to methanolic extracts of *E. globulus* showing high ZOI when compared with all other four plants.

All the pathogens except *Klebsiella* were susceptible to methanolic extracts of *H. sauveolens*. The maximum ZOI was 14 mm against *E. faecalis*. In the plant extracts from industrially polluted *Hiptis*, all the pathogens except *C. albicans* and *K. pneumonia* were susceptible to its extracts like the natural one where it shows 16 mm ZOI against *Enterococcus pneumonia* more than the natural one.

R. communis showed less antimicrobial activity. Only *B. cereus* and *E. pneumonia* are mainly susceptible. All others resisted or activity is insignificant. *R. communis* (natural) showed antimicrobial activity against one pathogen (*B. cereus*). The zone of inhibition was 11 mm. *R. communis* (polluted) showed antimicrobial activity against four pathogens (*S. aureus, B. subtilis, E. faecalis,* and *B. cereus*). The zone of inhibition was found between 7 and 10 mm. Hexane extracts of polluted plants showed 19 mm ZOI against *E. faecalis*.

T. cordifolia showed antimicrobial activity against all except *Shigella, Klebsiella,* and *E. coli*. The maximum ZOI showed against *B. cereus* 11 mm in chloroform of natural extracts and 17 mm of industrially polluted extracts. The most susceptible microorganisms in my study for plant extract in descending order were *B. cereus, S. aureus,* and *E. faecalis*.

The highest degree of antimicrobial activity was shown by *E. globulus* and had the highest ZOI at 20 mm among all the plants and *R. communis* having 5 mm had the minimum ZOI. The antimicrobial activity of both plants grown in polluted and natural conditions showed more similar activity where *A. vasica* and *E. globulus* grown in natural conditions showed better activity than plants grown in industrial polluted and *H. suaveolens, R. communis,* and *T. cordifolia* showed higher activity than plants grown in natural conditions.

From the MIC assays of 10 plant extracts, four plant extracts showed antimicrobial activities at minute quantities, 10 to 20 mg/ml concentration, as shown whereas a few plant extracts did not show any inhibitory effect in one or another bacterial and fungal species. The largest zone of inhibition belongs to *A. vasica* in both polluted and naturally grown extracts against *C.*

albicans, E. globulus, R. communis, and *T. cordifolia* against *B. cereus* and *H. sauveolens* against *E. faecalis* in all microbial studies.

The present study was designed to obtain information on the antimicrobial effect of 10 plant extracts on certain plant pathogenic microorganisms. The well diffusion/cup plate method was used in this study since it was found to be better than the disc diffusion method. All the medicinal plant extracts showed antimicrobial activity against the selected pathogens.

Hexane extract and chloroform extracts showed much lower or no antimicrobial activity compared with methanolic extracts. This may be due to little diffusion properties of these extracts in the agar or because fresh plants contain active substances which may be affected or removed by the steps of extraction methods. The methanolic extracts of all the medicinal plants screened exhibited greater antimicrobial activity. The antimicrobial action of methanolic extracts is due to compounds such as thiocyanate, nitrate, chloride, and sulphates beside other high-polarity soluble compounds which are naturally occurring in most plant materials [71].

This study showed that plant extracts were effective against the three Gram-positive strains (*S. aureus, B. subtilis,* and *B. cereus*) but no activity was observed against Gram-negative bacteria (*K. pneumonia, E. coli,* and *S. boydii*). This is consistent with previous studies reporting that Gram-negative bacteria are more resistant to antimicrobials than Gram-positive microorganisms due to their outer lipopolysaccharide membrane [72].

The presence of one or more of the secondary metabolites in my study indicated that the antibacterial activity was due to these active compounds present in different parts of the tested plants. The Gram-positive bacteria were slightly more susceptible to the extracts and showed greater inhibition zone than the Gram-negative bacteria, which in recent years have widely been reported in the literature [73].

Available reports tend to show that the secondary metabolites such as alkaloids, flavonoids, tannins, and other compounds of phenolic nature are responsible for the antimicrobial activities in higher plants [74]. The most studied chemical component in *A. vasica* is bitter quinazoline. The alkaloid vascine due to which the antimicrobial activity is seen [75]. The results provided evidence that *Hyptis* is indeed a potential source of natural antioxidant and antimicrobial agents. The antimicrobial activity could be due to the active chemical components savenine, alfa triterpines, 1–8 cinotene, cineole, and bita caryophyllene [76]. The results from *E. globulus* are promising and much higher than the earlier works [77]. The *Eucalyptus* antimicrobial activity is due to the active compound terpines.

The therapeutic activity of *R. communis* could be due to the recin chemical compound which is present and it also used experimentally in anticancer medicine [78]. The results indicated that the extracts of *R. communis* showed antibacterial activity, mainly against the Gram-negative bacteria (*E. coli*). The phytochemical components of *R. communis* have been established in previous studies and these include tannins, saponins, alkaloids, carbohydrates, phenols, flavonoids, sterols, and resins [79]. Several studies have linked the presence of these bioactive compounds in plant materials to antibacterial activity.

The antimicrobial activity of *T. cordifolia* is due to clerodane-derived diterpinoids, which comprise a large class of natural products with a wide range of biological activities [80]. The

http://dx.doi.org/10.5772/61891

plants *E. globulus* and *T. cordifolia* showed highest antimicrobial and high concentration of phenols and flavonoids are selected to work upon MCF-7 breast cancer cell lines for its anticancer activity. The difference in ZOI can be due to the environmental differences. The differences between minimum and maximum ZOI could also be attributed to the effects of Gram-positive and Gram-negative bacteria.

Among polluted and naturally grown plants, the plants grown in polluted areas showed more zones of inhibition than that of plants grown in natural conditions. Except for *A. vasica,* all four plants (*E. globulus, H. suaveolens, R. communis,* and *T. cordifolia*) grown in polluted areas showed zones of inhibition in more than four pathogens compared with plants grown in natural areas. Almost all five plants showed antimicrobial activity against *B. cereus* and zones of inhibition varied between 7 and 20 mm.

The phytochemically quantitative data revealed that the flavonoid and phenolic concentrations are higher in pollutant plants when compared to the control plants. Because phytochemicals could either have antioxidant or hormone-like actions for treating health condition including cancer, heart disease, diabetes, high blood pressure, and for preventing the formation of carcinogens on their target tissues. Flavonoids have been found to be antimicrobial substances against a wide array of microorganisms in vitro [81]. The plants studied here can be seen as a potential source of useful drugs. Further studies are to be investigated in order to isolate, identify, characterize, and elucidate the structure of bioactive compounds.

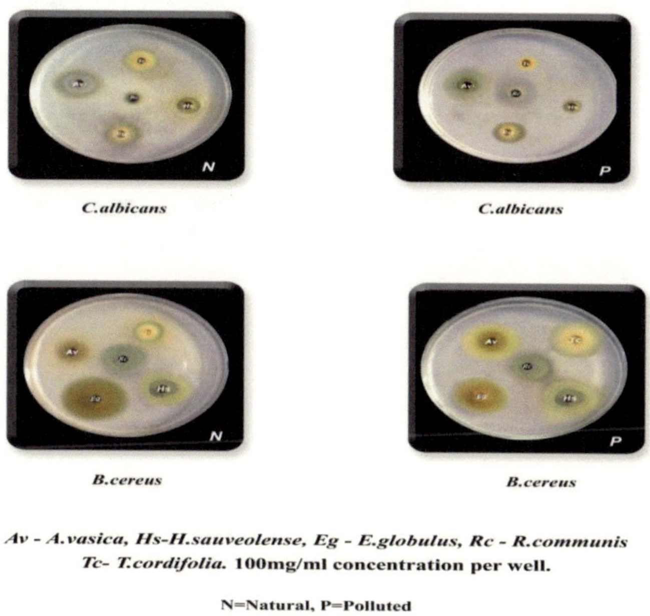

Plate 4. Antimicrobal Activity of Different Methanolic Plant Extracts against *C. albicans & B. cereus*

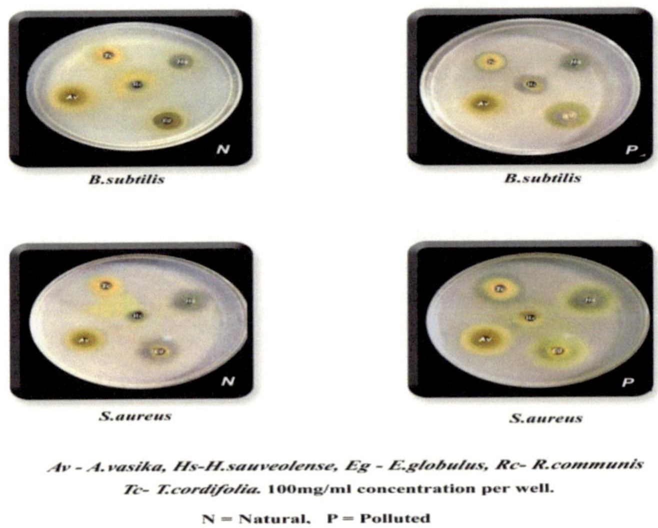

Plate 5. Antimicrobal Activity of Different Methanolic Plant Extracts against *B. subtilis & S. aureus*

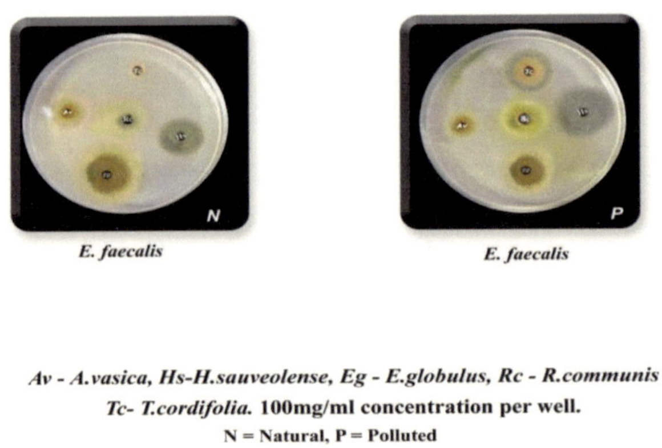

Plate 6. Antimicrobal Activity of Different Methanolic Plant Extracts against *E-faecalis*

4.3.1. The comparison/correlation between the result of phytochemical analysis and antimicrobial activity

The results showed that the phytochemical analysis is inconsistent with the antimicrobial activity that is seen in the same plants, namely, *H. suaveolens, Eucalyptus, Ricinus,* and *Tinospora* of the polluted areas which in turn showed increased phenolic and flavonoid content. The overall results and observations indicated that the plants that contained high metal concentrations tend to produce high amounts and high concentrations of phytochemicals, and this in turn resulted in the antimicrobial activity of the plants in coordination with the phytochemical analysis.

In support of these observations is the antimicrobial activity of the same four plants, *E. globulus*, *H. suoveolens*, *T. cordifolia*, and *R. communis*, which showed a zone of inhibition. The order of high total phenolic content was found to be 298.4, 283.6, 279.4, and 80 μg/mg in *H. suoveolens* (polluted), *T. cordifolia* (polluted), *E. globulus* (polluted), and *R. communis* (polluted), respectively. Similarly, the flavonoids order of high content was 33.3, 16.1, 13.6, and 9.9 mg/g in *H. suoveolens* (polluted), *E. globulus* (polluted), *R. communis* (polluted), and *T. cordifolia* (polluted), respectively. But in *E. globulus* (natural), the high concentrations of flavonoids are seen at 21.4 mg/g than polluted.

4.4. Anticancer activity

The cytotoxic effects of the methanolic crude extracts of *E. globulus* and *T. cordifolia* were evaluated on MCF-7 breast cancer cell lines by microculture XTT assay. The multiple concentrations of methanolic extracts from *E. globulus* and *T. cordifolia* were used and effective doses were calculated from the dose–response curve. The results of cytotoxicity evaluated against MCF-7 using extracts at different concentrations (6.25, 1.5, 25, 50, 100, and 200 μg/ml) (Table 15). The methanol extracts of *E. globulus* and *T. cordifolia* exhibited cytotoxic effects on MCF-7 cell lines were confirmed by XTT assay.

Conc (μg/ml)	OD of STD (Tamoxifen) at 490 nm	% CS	% CI	OD of E.g (N) At 490 nm	% CS	% CI	OD of E.g (P) at 490 nm	% CS	% CI	OD of T.c (N) at 490 nm	% CS	% CI
6.25	0.423	83.8	16.2	0.492	98.9	1.1	0.488	98	2	0.485	97.4	2.6
12.5	0.322	61.7	38.3	0.473	94.7	5.3	0.462	92.3	7.7	0.468	93.7	6.3
25	0.246	45.1	54.9	0.386	75.7	24.3	0.352	68.3	31.7	0.361	70.2	29.8
50	0.179	30.4	69.6	0.365	71.1	28.9	0.315	60.2	39.8	0.331	63.7	36.3
100	0.095	12	87	0.272	50.8	49.2	0.285	53.6	46.4	0.288	54.3	45.7
200	0.058	3.9	96.1	0.234	42.5	57.5	0.222	39.8	60.2	0.257	47.5	52.5

Conc (μg/ml)	OD of T.c(P) STD at 490mm	% CS	% CI	OD of E.g + T.c (N) at 490 nm	% CS	% CI	OD of E.g (P) +T.c (P) at 490 nm	% CS	% CI
6.25	0.495	99.6	0.4	0.485	97.4	2.6	0.474	95	5
12.5	0.486	97.6	2.4	0.444	88.4	11.6	0.462	92.3	7.6
25	0.426	84.5	15.5	0.356	69.1	30.9	0.382	74.8	25.2
50	0.372	72.6	27.4	0.257	47.5	52.5	0.276	51.6	48.4
100	0.269	50.1	49.9	0.142	22.3	77.7	0.176	29.8	70.2
200	0.215	38.3	61.7	0.113	16	84	0.126	18.8	81.2

Blank = 0.040, Control = 0.497

E.g = *E. globulus*, T.c = *T. cordifolia*. N = natural, P = polluted.

Table 15. Dose–response of *E. globulus and T. cordifolia on* MCF-7 cell line

At the final tested concentration (200 μg/ml), the cytotoxicity of *E. globulus* grown in natural and polluted areas was 57.5% and 60.2%, respectively. The effects were dose-dependent and based on a dose–response curve, IC_{50} values were determined (Table 16). The methanol extracts of *E. globulus* exhibited antiproliferative effects on both cell lines with IC_{50} values of 145.85 and 136.53 μg/ml, respectively. From these results, it is evident that the effect of *E. globulus* extract from natural areas showed less cytotoxicity than the *E. globulus* from polluted areas. The cytotoxicity of the crude extracts from both are halfway ranging between 50% and 60% to reach the results of control tamoxifen, where it was 96.1%.

Plant	E.g(N)	E.g(P)	T.c(N)	T.c(P)	E.g(N)+T.c(N)	E.g(P)+T.c(P)
IC_{50}	145.85 μg/ml	136.53 μg/ml	156.95 μg/ml	139.91 μg/ml	82.400 μg/ml	91.980 μg/ml
Slope	0.27773134	0.26371002	0.23139161	0.32012509	0.40436674	0.39459844
Correlation coefficient	0.907716280	0.86551911	0.8376033	0.9425528	0.88480409	0.90949691
Intercept	9.49054726	13.9940299	13.681592	5.20845771	16.6800995	13.7044776

E.g = E. globulus, T.c = T. cordifolia. N = natural P = polluted.

Table 16. The IC_{50} values of plant extracts used against MCF-7 cell lines

4.4.1. The cytotoxic effect of methanolic extracts of T. cordifolia on MCF-7 breast cancer cell line by XTT assay

At the final concentration of 200 μg/ml the cytotoxicity of *T. cordifolia* grown in natural and polluted areas were 52.5% and 61.7% respectively based on the dose–response curve IC_{50} values were determined (Table 16). The plant extracts exhibited high antiproliferative effect on MCF-7 cell lines with IC_{50} values of 156.95 and 139.91 μg/ml, respectively. And like in the case of *E. globulus*, the cytotoxicity is less in *T. cordifolia* natural areas than that of polluted areas.

4.4.2. The cytotoxic effect of combined extracts of E. globulus and T. cordifolia from natural and polluted sources on MCF-7 cell lines

The cytotoxic effect of combined samples proved better results in comparison with the individual samples. The combined samples of *E. globulus* and *T. cordifolia* natural areas showed final concentrations of 200 μg/ml, 84% of cell inhibition having IC_{50} value 81.400 μg/ml and the *E. globulus* and *T. cordifolia* polluted areas showed 81.2% of cell inhibition IC_{50} value 91.980 μg/ml (Tables 15 and 16).

Here, contrary to the individual samples, the cytotoxicity exhibited by the combined extract of plants grown in polluted areas were less than that of natural extracts. The cytotoxicity results were also promising as the cytotoxicity of the combined extracts almost neared substituting the control tamoxifen results of 96.1% at the final concentration.

4.4.3. Evaluation of morphological changes of MCF-7 cell lines upon treatment with extracts

The morphological changes of MCF-7 cell lines treated with extracts from plants grown in both polluted and natural resources were observed under phase contract microscope. The cells indicated most prominent effect after exposure to the extracts of *E. globulus* and *T. cordifolia* from polluted areas and their combined extracts compared with that of individual extracts of *E. globulus* and *T. cordifolia* from natural areas. In the combined sample extracts, 40% to 50% of the cells showed membrane blebbing (demonstrated with small protrusions of the membrane) and ballooning were apparent in the cells.

Cells also showed extensive vacuolation in the cytoplasm, indicating autophagy-like mechanism of cell death. Autophagosome-like structures were clearly seen in the cells treated with extract. At the highest concentration (200 μg/ml) the cells became rounder, shrunken, and showed signs of detachment from the surface of the wells denoting cell death.

In the present study, anticancer activity of extracts of indigenous medicinal plants *E. globulus* and *T. cordifolia* grown in polluted and natural sources were investigated against human breast cancer cells MCF-7, whereas tamoxifen was used as experimental controls. A methodical evaluation of cytotoxicity effects revealed that the individual methanolic extract of *E. globulus* and *T. cordifolia* polluted and natural areas and their combined samples and tamoxifen showed dose-dependent cytotoxicity against MCF-7 cell lines. The IC_{50} values of combined plant extracts were found to be less than 100 μg/ml, indicating potent cytotoxic effects on breast cancer cell lines and further potential of these extracts for the isolation of biologically active phytochemicals. Most anticancer drugs are designed to eliminate rapidly proliferating cancerous cells and therefore they show cytotoxicity and induce apoptosis in cancer cells.

The phytochemical analysis of my study observed the presence of a large number of bioactive compounds in the methanolic extracts of these plants including terpenoids, alkaloids, phenols, and flavonoids, which exhibit various biological activities. These compounds hold great potential as drugs and are widely accepted among the public. This investigation provides evidence for cytotoxicity in MG(F)-7, which may be due to existing phytochemicals in the extract as mentioned previously. The sensitivities of cancer cells to cell death by flavonoids are in accordance with findings from previous reports in the literature. In another study, the presence of alkaloids with flavonoids in Onobishirta was reported expressing superior activity against cancer cells.

Our results are on par with the results that the phytochemicals present in *T. cordifolia* have potent cytotoxic and anticancer potential against MCF-7 cell lines [82]. Cancer cell lines used in the study exhibited differential sensitivity towards different plant extracts. The differential behavior of cell lines may be due to the different molecular characteristics of these cells. The present study clearly indicates that *T. cordifolia* extracts are very active against human breast cancer cell lines.

Polyphenols have been shown to possess antimutagenic and antimalignant effects. Moreover, flavonoids have a chemopreventive role in cancer through their effects on signal transduction in cell proliferation and angiogenesis.

MCF-7 breast cancer cell lines.

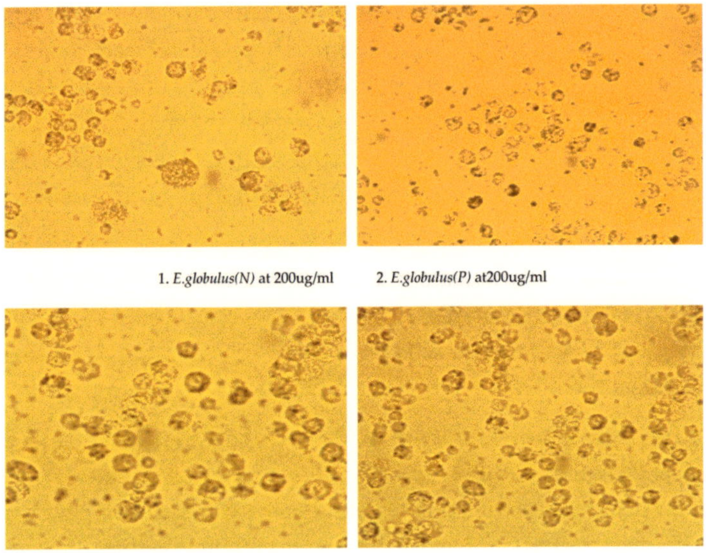

1. *E.globulus(N)* at 200ug/ml 2. *E.globulus(P)* at200ug/ml

3. *T.cordifolia(N)* at 200ug/ml 4. *T.cordifolia(P)* at 200ug/ml

N= NATURAL P= POLLUTED

Plate 7. Anticancer activity of methanolic crude plant extracts against MCF-7 breast cancer cell lines.

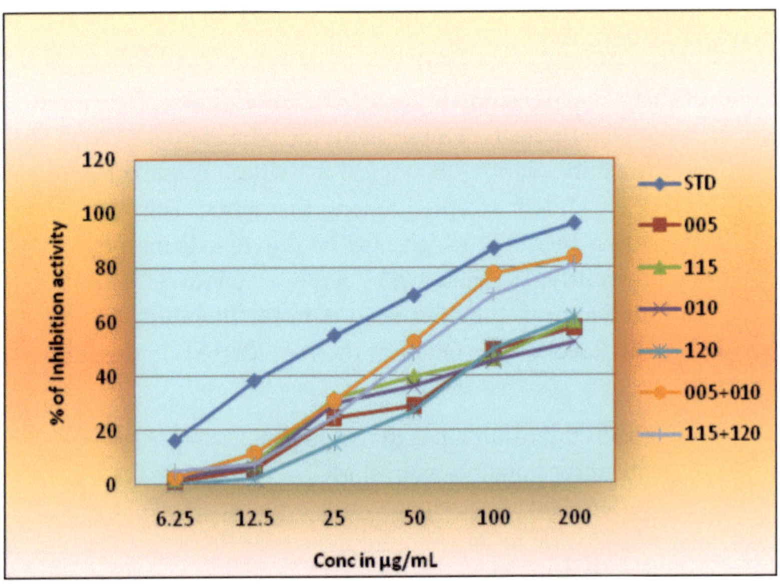

E.g=Eucalyptus globulus(N)=005, T.c=Tinospora cordifolia(N)=010,
E.g=Eucalyptus globulus(P)=II5, T.c=Tinospora cordifolia(P)=120, N=Natural, P=Polluted

Figure 8. Anticancer activity of *E. globulus* and *T. cordifolia* plant extracts on MCF-7 breast cancer cell lines.

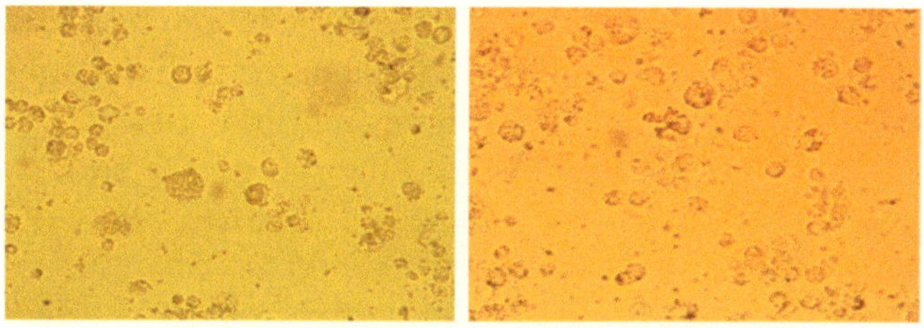

5. *E.globulus* (N)+*T.c (N)* at 200ug/ml   6. *E.globulus(P)+T.c(P)* at200ug/ml

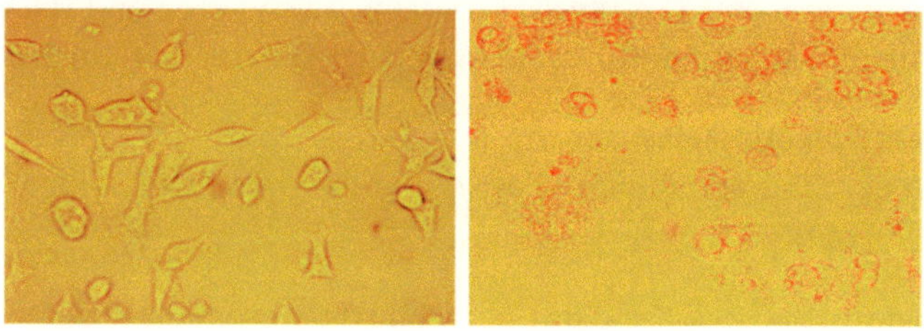

7. MCF-7 Untreated   8. Tamoxifen treated MCF-7

N= NATURAL   P= POLLUTED

Plate 8. Anticancer activity of methanolic crude plant extracts against MCF-7 breast cancer cell lines.

The cytotoxic and antitumor properties of the extract may be due to presence of these compounds have shown very high efficacy in *T. cordifolia* extracts against Dalton lymphoma ascites (DLA) tumor model in Swiss albino mice in terms of survival as well as tumor volume control [82]. However, the exact mechanism is not clear. Available evidence suggests that DNA damage, inhibition of topoisomerase II, decline in clonogenecity and glutathione-S-transferase activity, activation of tumor associated macrophage, increase in lipid peroxidation, and LDH release are probable mechanisms behind the cytotoxic activity [83]. The arabinogalactan present in aqueous extracts of guduchi stem have also been shown to produce immunological activity. Many of the compounds mentioned above have been reported to be cytotoxic.

In this study the findings show there is much relationship between anticancer activity and phenolic composition. The extract of polluted plants that showed high anticancer activity also showed high phenolic composition. The finding suggests that the plants grown under polluted conditions reduced the number of viable cells compared with that of plants grown under natural conditions. As the geochemical analysis ruled out the toxicity of heavy metals in these plants as their concentrations fell below the permissible limits and the scope of using plants under abiotic stress and the taboo of avoiding these medicinal plants could be altered by further studies in these areas.

5. Summary and conclusion

The present research work "*Phytopharmaceutical studies on selected medicinal plants subjected to abiotic elicitation (stress) in an industrial area of Malkapuram, Visakhapatnam district of Andhra*

Pradesh" was undertaken to study the effect of industrial pollution on selected medicinal plants that were thriving well and growing luxuriantly compared with the same plants grown in natural or less polluted conditions. Malkapuram industrial area in Visakhapatnam was selected as the polluted region and Paderu, the hilly and agency area, was selected as the natural or less polluted region. To fulfill the aims and objectives, I have carried out the work in six phases:

i. The plants, namely, *A. vasica* (Nees), *E. globulus* (Labill), *H. sauveolens* (L.) Poit, *R. communis* (Linn.), and *T. cordifolia* (Miers) were collected and selected for my study from industrial areas and the same from natural areas that are grown luxuriantly.

ii. To check out abiotic stress, namely, metal stress, the metal analysis of selected plants grown in both industrial/natural areas and the soil in which the plants were grown was carried out.

iii. Subsequently, to check the effect of metal stress on phytochemicals, the qualitative and quantitative analysis of selected plants and the correlation between metal analysis and phytochemicals was studied.

iv. To see the effect of phytochemicals, the antimicrobial activity of the same plants was done using 8 pathogens.

v. *E. globulus* (Labill) and *T. cordifolia* (Miers), two plants that showed high concentrations of phenols and flavonoids as well as better antimicrobial activity were checked out for their anticancer activity against MCF-7 breast cancer cell lines.

vi. The entire data of my research work was analyzed statistically by applying SPSS.

No comparative studies of these medicinal plants under abiotic stress have been carried out so far. Pollution and its effect on flora and fauna is a global issue today. The metal analysis, phytochemical, antimicrobial, and anticancer activities of medicinal plants under abiotic stress is rare and scanty. The salient findings of the present study are furnished below.

1. The metal analysis of soils from an industrially polluted area of Malkapuram and a natural area revealed that the metal concentration is higher in the industrially polluted area compared with that of natural soils collected from the Paderu region of Visakhapatnam district and the heavy metal concentrations in both areas are below the regulatory limits of soil adopted from the U.S. EPA (1993).

2. The metal analysis of plants resulted in high metal concentrations in industrial polluted plants than that of plants grown in natural conditions, and heavy metal concentrations falling below the permissible limits of WHO/FAO (1984). It is also evident even though the soils contained high concentrations of metals, that the plants did not contain the same as they absorbed selectively based on different factors.

3. The preliminary phytochemical analysis results were in positive correlation with the metal analysis where the industrial polluted methanolic extracts contained more

http://dx.doi.org/10.5772/61891

phytochemicals in comparison with the methanolic extracts of plants grown in natural areas.

4. The total phenolics concentration showed a significant increase in the plants grown in polluted conditions and, in some, 2- to 3-fold increases than the plants from natural areas. The flavonoid concentrations are at par with phenolics but with less significance.

5. The antimicrobial activity of the methanolic plant extracts that contained a greater degree of concentration of phenolics and flavonoids showed a higher percentage of activity. The methanolic extract of *E. globulus* grown in industrial polluted area having 100% activity against pathogens followed by *A. vasica* Nees and *H. sauvelens* (L.) from polluted areas.

6. The anticancer activity of *E. globulus and T. cordifolia* were selected from five plants with a high concentration of phenols and flavonoids confirmed the activity of MCF-7 breast cancer cell lines. At 200 μg/ml, the methanolic extracts of plants from polluted areas showed 57%–67% cell inhibition and combined extracts showed 81%–84% of cell inhibition of MCF-7 breast cancer cell lines having IC_{50} values below 100 μg/ml, which gives scope and way for further work in this area.

7. The statistical analysis carried out for the entire data from my results by using SPSS has further strengthened the findings of my work.

It is therefore through my findings that the following suggestions and conclusions are proposed:

1. The abiotic stress on plants grown in industrial polluted area triggered increased productivity of phytochemicals that lead to promising antimicrobial and anticancer activity of methanolic plant extracts, paving a definite way for pharmaceutical industries.

2. To exploit the plants under stress for preparations of novel drugs by extracting larger quantities of therapeutic chemicals to meet the needs of a growing population with less usage of plant dry mass.

3. As all the heavy metal concentrations fell below the permissible limits of FAO/WHO in the plants from polluted areas and as it showed significant increase in the phenols and flavonoids, it is recommended that pharmaceutical industries exploit plants under stress for therapeutic measures than the plants from natural areas after a strict screening for toxic elements.

4. As 80%–90% of the population depends on herbal medicine due to its' cost, side effects, and drug resistance, these plants could be further screened for any toxicity and made available for therapeutic uses.

5. The anticancer findings suggested that the plants grown under polluted conditions reduced the number of viable cells than that of plants grown under natural conditions. As the geochemical analysis ruled out the toxicity of heavy metals in these plants as their concentrations fell below permissible limits and the scope of using plants under abiotic stress and the taboo of avoiding these medicinal plants could be altered by further studies in these areas.

6. As the percentage of cell inhibition by *E. globulus* and *T. cordifolia* are close to the percentage of antibiotic tamoxifen, it could be further proposed to test the efficacy of its anticancer activity with live cells.

Author details

Sr. Prema Kumari Jonnada[1], Louis Jesudas[2] and Varaprasad Bobbarala[3*]

*Address all correspondence to: varaprasad.bobbarala@gmail.com

1 St. Ann's College for Woman, Malkapuram, Visakhapatnam, Andhra Pradesh, India

2 Department of Plant Biology and Plant Biotechnology, St. Xavier's College (Affiliated to MS University) Palayamkottai, Nellai, Tamil Nadu, India

3 Scientific Consultant, Sreenivasa Nagar, Kancharapalem, Visakhapatnam, Andhra Pradesh, India

References

[1] Samata, S. 2011. Impacts of Government Policies on Sustenance of Tribal People in Visakhapatnam. Visakhapatnam: Mittal Publications.

[2] Karthikeyan, A., Shanthi, V., Nagasathaya, A. 2009. Preliminary phytochemical and antimicrobacterial screening of crude extract of the leaf of *Adhatoda vasica* L. *International Journal of Green Pharmacy* 78–80.

[3] Ekwenye, U.N., E.N. 2005. Antibacterial activity of ginger (*Zingiber officials* Roscoe) and garlic (*Allium sativum* L.) extracts on *Escherichia coli* and *Salmonella typhi*. *Journal of Molecular Medicine and Advanced Science* 1(4): 411–416, 8.

[4] Ncube, N.S., Afolayan, A. Okoh A.L. 2008. Assessment techniques ofantimicrobial properties of natural compounds of plant origin: current methods and future trends. *African Journal of Biotechnology* 7(12): 1797–1806.

[5] Masorini, R. 1987. Elemental investigation of *Momordica charantia* Linn. and *Syziginm jambolana* Linn. using atomic absorption spectrophotometer. *Bulletin of the World Health Organization* 40:305.

[6] Chaudhary, R., Jahan, S., Goyal, P.K. 2008. Chemopreventive potential of an Indian medicinal plant (*Tinospora cordifolia*) on skin carcinogenesis in mice. *Journal of Environmental Pathology, Toxicology, and Oncology* 27(3): 233–243.

[7] Sahito, S., Kazi, T.G., J.M. 2008. Elemental investigation of *Momordica charantia* Linn. and *Syngium jambolana* Linn. using atomic absorption spectrophotometer. *The Nucleus* 39: 49–54.

[8] Baker, J.T. 1995. Natural product drug discovery and development. New perspective on international collaboration. *Journal of Natural Product* 58: 1325–1357.

[9] Khanna, P. 1995. Off site emergency preparedness plan for Visakhapatnam district. *Area Risk Assessment* 1: 189–190, –8.

[10] Nies, P. 1999. Microbial heavy metal resistance. *Applied Microbiology Biotechnology* 51, 732–750, –9.

[11] Dewick, P. 1996. Tumor inhibition from plants. *Tease and Evans.*

[12] Phillipson, J.W. 1996. Plants with antiprotozoal activity. *Tease and Evans, Pharmacognosy*. London: WB Saunders Company.

[13] Arunkumar, S.M. 2009. Analysis of phytochemical constituents and antimicrobial activities of *Aloe vera* L. against clinical pathogens. *World Journal of Agricultural Science* 5(5): 572–576.

[14] Mojab, F., Kamalinejad, M., Ghaderi, N., Vanidipour, H.R. 2003. Phytochemicals screening of some species of Iranian plants. *Iranian Journal of Pharmaceutical Research* 3: 77–82.

[15] Parekh, J., Chanda, S. 2008. Phytochemical screening of some plants from western region of India. *Plant Archives* 8: 657–662.

[16] Ministry of Environment and Forest. 1995. Offside emerging preparedness plan for Visakhapatnam district. *Area Risk Assesment* 1: 188. –13.

[17] Padal, S.B., Prayaga Murty, P., Srinivasa Rao, D., Venkaiah, M. 2010. Ethnomedicinal plants from Paderu division of Visakhapatnam district. *Journal of Phytology* 2(8): 70–91. –14.

[18] Drew, M. 1998. Stress physiology. In: *Plant Physiology,* Taiz, L., Zeiger, E., editors. –15.

[19] Perez-Balibrea, S., Moreno, D.A., and Garcia-Viguera, C. 2008. Influence of light on health-promoting phytochemicals of broccoli sprouts. *Journal of Science, Food and Agriculture* 88, 904–910. –16.

[20] Gershenzon, J. 1998. Plant defenses: surface protection and secondary metabolites. In: *Plant Physiology*. Taiz, L., Zeiger, E., editors. Sunderland, MA: The Sinauer Associates, Inc. p. 347–376. –17.

[21] Nasim, S.A., and Dhir, B. 2010. Heavy metals alter the potency of medicinal plants. *Reviews of Environmental Contamination and Toxicology* 203: 139–149. –18.

[22] Michalak, A. 2006. Phenolic compounds and their antioxidant activity in plants growing under heavy metal stress. *Polish Journal of Environmental Studies* 15: 523–530. –19.

[23] King, H., A.R. 1998. Global burden of diabetes 1995–2025. Prevalence, numberical estimates, and projections. *Diabetes Care*, 129–134.

[24] Rajurkar, N.S., and Perdeshi, B.M. 1997. *Applied Radiation and Isotopes* 48: 1059, 15.

[25] Kamath, R, Mahajan, K.S., Ashok, L., Sanal, T.S. 2013. A study on risk factors of breast cancer among patients attending the tertiary care hospital in Udupi district. *Indian Journal of Community Medicine* 38:95–99.

[26] Ramachandra Reddy, K. 2011. Cancer Statistics. Dept. of Epidemiology and Biostatistics, Kidwai Memorial Institute of Oncology. –25.

[27] World Health Organization (WHO) 2010. International Agency for Research on Cancer, press release, 28 March, 2010. –26.

[28] Times of India. 2012. Cancer statistics in Indian women. Oct 21–27.

[29] Gamble, J.S. 1915–1936. Flora of the Presidency of Madras. Adlard & Sons Ltd., London, 37.

[30] Subba Rao, G.V. 1977. Flora of Visakhapatnam district, Andhra Pradesh. *Bulletin of the Botanical Survey of India* 19:122–126. –38.

[31] Seshagiri, R.R., Harasreeramulu, S. 1986. Flora of Srikakulam District, Andhra Pradesh, India. Ed. Meerut: Indian Botanical Society. 640 pp. –39.

[32] Gamble, J.S. 2004. Flora of the presidency of Madras. Bishen Singh Mahendra Pal Singh, ed. 1, pp. lxiv + 2017.

[33] Gamble, J.S. 2005. Flora of the presidency of Madras. Bishen Singh Mahendra Pal Singh, ed. 1, pp. lxiv + 2017.

[34] Brindha, P., Sasikala, B., and Purushothaman, K.K. 1981. Pharmacognostic studies on Merugan kilzhangu. BMEBR 3(1): 84–96. –40.

[35] Swain, T., Hillis, W.E. 1959. The phenolic constituents of *Prunus domestica*. I. The quantitative analysis of phenolic constituents. *Journal of the Science of Food and Agriculture* 10(1): 63–68 –41.

[36] Singleton, V.L., and Rossi, J.A. 1965. Calorimetry of total phenolics with phasphomolybdic and phaphotungestic acid reagents. *American Journal of Enology and Viticulture* 16:144–158. –42.

[37] Murray, S.S., Chappell, J.H., Kenter, A.T., Kraft, R.P., Meehan, G.R., and M.V. Zombeck. 1995. *Proceedings of SPIE* 3356:974. –43.

[38] Olurinola, P.F., and Ibrahim, Y.K. 1991. Comparative microbial contamination levels in wet granulation and direct compression methods of tablet production, *Pharmaceutica Acta Helvetiae* 66:298–301.

[39] Scudiero, D.A., Shoemaker, R.H., Paull, K.D., Monks, A., Tierney, S., Nofziger, T.H., Currens, M.J., Seniff, D., Boyd, M.R. 1988. Evaluation of a soluble tetrazolium/formazan assay for cell growth and drug sensitivity in culture using human and other tumor cell lines. *Cancer Research* 48:4827–4833.

[40] Cataldo, D.A., and Wildung, R.E. 1978. Soil and plant factors influencing the accumulation of heavy metals by plants. *Environmental Health Perspectives* 27: 149–159.

[41] Domy, C. Adriane. 2001. Trace Elements in Terrestrial Environment–Biogeochemistry, Bioavailability and Risks of Metals. 2nd ed., University of Georgia, USA. –46.

[42] Brian, J. Alloway. 2013. Heavy metals in soils. 3rd ed., Springer Science + Business Media Dordrecht, UK. –47.

[43] U.S. EPA. 1996. Report: Recent Developments for *In situ* Treatment of Metals-Contaminated Soils. U.S. Environmental Protection Agency, Office of Solid Waste and Emergency Response. –48.

[44] Cragg, G.M., Newman, D.J. 2001. Natural product drug discovery in the next millennium. *Pharmaceutical Biology* 39: 8–17, –49.

[45] Khan, S.A., Ahmad, I., Mohajir, M.S. 2006. Evaluation of mineral content of some edible medicinal plants. *Pakistan Journal of Pharmaceutical Sciences* 19(2): 141–148.

[46] Margo, A., Diallo, I.D., Byo, R., and Paudren, B.S. 2005. Determination of some toxic and essential metal ions in medicinal edible plants from Mali. *Journal of Agricultural and Food Chemistry* 53: 2316–2321. –50.

[47] Haffland, E., Kuyper, T.W., Wallander, H., et al. 2004. The role of fungi in weathering. *Frontiers in Ecology and the Environment* 2: 258–264. –51.

[48] FAO/WHO. 1984. Contaminants. In Codex Alimentarius, vol. XVII, ed. 1. FAO/WHO, Codex Alimentarius Commision, Rome, –56.

[49] Gupta, U. 1975. *Copper in the Environment*. J. O. Nariago, ed., John Wiley and Sons, New York, 255.

[50] Shumacher, M., Bosque, M.A., and Domingo, J.L., Carbella, J. 1991. *Bulletin of Environmental Contamination and Toxicology* 46: 320.

[51] Grath, S.P., and Smith, S. 1990. *Chromium and Nickel in Heavy Metals in Soils*. B.J. Alloway, ed. Blackie: Glasgow, 125.

[52] Gorbanova, V.A. 2004. *Journal of Environmental Protection and Ecology* 5(2): 281, –61.

[53] Nath, R. 1986. *Biological and Health Effects Interprint*. India, –63.

[54] Smith, L.A., Means, J.L., Chen, A. 1995. *Remedial Options for Metals-Contaminated Site*. Lewis Publishers, Boca Raton, FL, USA, –65.

[55] Pendias, A.K., and Pendias, H. 1992. Trace elements in soils and plants. 2nd ed., Boca Raton, FL: CRC Press, 365.

[56] Huheey, J.E., Ellen Keiter, A., Richard Keiter, L. Okhil, K. 2007. Medhi inorganic chemistry. *Principles of Sructure and Reactivity* (Pearson Edu). 751–758.

[57] Yadav, S.K. 2010. Heavy metals toxicity in plants: An overview on the role of glutathione and phytochelatins in heavy metal stress tolerance of plants. *South African Journal of Botany* 76:16–179.

[58] Yadav, S.K. 2010. Heavy metals toxicity in plants: An overview on the role of glutathione and phytochelatins in heavy metal stress tolerance of plants. *South African Journal of Botany* 76:16–179.

[59] Arvind Kumar Sharma, Amit Kumar, Sharad Kumar Yadav, and Anu Rahal. 2014. Studies on antimicrobial and immunomodulatory effects of hot aqueous extract of *Acacia nilotica* L. leaves against common veterinary pathogens. *Veterinary Medicine International* 9 pp., 2014. doi:10.1155/2014/747042-71.

[60] Nithya, T.G., Vidhya, V.G., Sangeetha, K., and Vimala Prakash. 2011. Phytochemical screening of a polyherb Vallarai chooranam. *International Journal of Drug Formulation and Research* 2: 294–301, –72.

[61] Venkatswamy, R., Doss, A., Sukumar, M., and Mubarack, H.M. 2010, Preliminary phytochemical screening and antimicrobial studies of *Lantana indica* Roxb. *Indian Journal of Pharmaceutical Sciences* 72(2): 229–231 –73.

[62] Daniel, V.N., Daniang, I.E. 2011. Phytochemical analysis and mineral elements composition of *Ocium sasilicum* obtained in Jos metropolis, Plateau State. *International Journal of Engineering & Technology* 06, –74.

[63] Mohammad Rahimi, Reza Farhadi, Mojib Salehi Balashahri. 2012. Effects of heavy metals on the medicinal plant. *International Journal of Agronomy and Plant Production* 3(4): 154–158, –75.

[64] Shariff, Z.U. 2001. *Modern Herbal Therapy for Common Ailments*. Nature Pharmacy Series, Volume 1, Spectrum Books Limited, Ibadan, Nigeria in Association with Safari Books (Export) Limited, United Kingdom, pp. 9–84, –76.

[65] Han, X., Shen, T., Lou, H. 2007. Dietry polyphenols and their biological significance. *International Journal of Molecular Sciences* 950–988, –78.

[66] Okwu, D.E., and Okwu, M.E. 2004. Chemical composition of *Spondias mombin* Linn. plant part. *Journal of Sustainable Agriculture and the Environment* 6(2): 140–147, –79.

[67] Antherden, L.M. 1969. *Textbook of Pharmaceutical Chemistry*, 8th ed., London: Oxford University Press, p. 813. –80.

[68] Harborne, J.B. 1996. *International Journal of Plant Biochemistry and Molecular Biology*. London: Elsevier Science Ltd. 43: 1325–1331, 43: 1076–1081, 44:107–111, –81.

[69] Theodora-Ioanna Lafka, Andriana E. Lazou, Vassilia J. Sinanoglou, and Evangelos S. Lazos. 2013. Phenolic extracts from wild olive leaves and their potential as edible oils antioxidants. *Foods* 2: 18–31.

[70] Zachariah, Vidya. 1986. *Flora of Srikakulam District, Andhra Pradesh, India*. Ed. Meerut: Indian Botanical Society. 640 pp. anad, Aleykutty, Jaykar, Halima 2012. Free radical scavenging and antibacterial activity of *Mirabilis jalapa* Linn. using in vitro models. *IRJP*, 3: (3).

[71] Darout, I., Cristy, A., Skaug, N., and P. Egeberg. 2000. Identification andquantification of some potentially antimicrobial anionic components in Miswak extract. *Indian Journal of Pharmacology* 32:11–14.

[72] Khan, M.A., D. Shahwar, N. Ahmad, Z. Khan, and M. Ajaib. 2009. Chemical constituents of *Carissa opaca* extracts and their evaluation as antioxidant and preservative in edible oils. *Asian Journal of Chemistry* 22(1): 379–388, –88.

[73] Jigna Parekh and Sumitra Chanda. 2006. Antibacterial and phytochemical studies on twelve species of Indian medicinal plants. *African Journal of Biomedical Research* 10: 175–181.

[74] Mishra, A., Kumar, S., Bhargava, A., Sharma, B. and Pandey, A.K. 2012 Studies on in vitro antioxidant and antistaphylococcal activities of some important medicinal plants. *Cellular and Molecular Biology* 57:16–25, –23.

[75] Lahiri, P.K., and Prahdan, S.N. 1964. Pharmacological investigation of vasicinol—an alkaloid from *Adhatoda vasica* Nees. *Indian Journal of Experimental Biology* 2: 219–223, –90.

[76] Witayapan Nantitanon, Sombat Chowwanapoonpohn, Siriporn Okonogi. 2007. Antioxidant and antimicrobial activities of *Hyptis suaveolens* essential oil. *Scientia Pharmaceutica* 75: 35–46.

[77] Bachir Raho, G., Benali, M. 2012. Antibacterial activity of the essential oils from the leaves of *Eucalyptus globulus* against *Escherichia coli* and *Staphylococcus aureus*. *Asian Pacific Journal of Tropical Biomedicine* 2(9): 739–742, –92.

[78] Chang, N., Kleinstreuer, P., Ceger, J., Hamm, B., Jones, L., Rinckel. 2014 Development of reverse T models for IVIVC of ER activity NICEATM-ICCVAM future Tox II 2013 poser albino mice. *eCAM* 4: 343–350, –93.

[79] Biswas, K.I., Chattopadhyay, A., Banerjee, Y.A., Bandopadhyay, U. 2002. Biological activities and medicinal properties of neem. *Current Science* 82: 1336–1345. –94.

[80] Oberlies, N.M., Burgess, J.P., Navarro, H.A., Pinos, R.E., Fairchild, C.R., Peterson, R.W., Soejatto, D.D., Famaworth, N.R., Kingdom, A.D., Wani, M.C., Wall, M.E. 2002.

Novel bioactive clerodane diterpenoids from the leaves and twigs of *Casearia sylvestris*. *Journal of Natural Products* 65: 95–99, –95.

[81] Marjorie, C. 1996. Plant products as antimicrobial agents. *Clinical Microbiology Reviews* 12:564–582.

[82] Amit Mishra, Shashank Kumar, Abhay K. Pandey. 2013. Scientific validation of the medicinal efficacy of *Tinospora cordifolia*. Dept of Biochemistry. University of Allahabad. Antioxidant potential of ethyl acetate extract/fractions of *Acacia auriculiformis*. *A. Cunn. Fod Chem.Toxicol*. 45: 1216–1223.

[83] Adhvaryu, M.R., Reddy, N., Parabia, M.H. 2007. Effects of four Indian medicinal herbs on isoniazid, rifampicin- and pyrazinamide-induced hepatic injury and immunosuppression in guinea pigs. *World Journal of Gastroenterology* 13(23): 199–205, –33.

[84] Jagetia, G.C., Rao, S.K. 2006. Evaluation of cytotoxic effects of dichloromethane extract of guduchi (*Tinospora cordifolia* Miers ex Hook F & Thoms) on cultured HeLa cells. *Evidence-Based Complementary and Alternative Medicine* 3(2): 267–272, –32.